Long-term Homeoprophylaxis Study in Children in North America: Part One and Part Two

Establishing Homeoprophylaxis as a Public Health Model

By
Kate Birch, RSHom(NA) CCH
Su Sandon, RPh, RSHom(NA) CCH, HMC
Sarah Damlo, C.Hom
Kim Lane, MD

Free and Healthy Children International

Dedication

To all children who invited your parents to look for another option
in disease prevention.

To all families looking to educate your children's immune systems
towards infectious contagious disease.

To all practitioners searching for data to expand your
understanding of homeoprophylaxis.

To all political leaders and doctors who are in the position to
regulate and apply public health models, may you consider there is
another way.

For the betterment of humanity: may we work together to preserve
the integrity of all children's immune systems in relation to
infectious disease and realize the benefits of immunological
education with regards to all aspects of human evolution.

Other books

For more information on homeopathy and homeoprophylaxis and the risks of vaccines we recommend these books:

1. **The Solution ~ Homeoprophylaxis: The Vaccine Alternative**. A Parent's Guide to Educating Your Child's Immune System. Kate Birch, RSHom(NA), CCH, CMT & Cilla Whatcott, HD(RHom), CCH.
2. **Vaccine Free Prevention and Treatment of Infectious Contagious Disease with Homeopathy**. A Manual for Practitioners and Consumers. Kate Birch, RSHom(NA), CCH, CMT.
3. **There is a Choice: Homeoprophylaxis**. An Appeal to Mothers. Cilla Whatcott, PhD, HD(RHom), CCH.
4. **The Complete Practitioners Manual of Homeoprophylaxis**. Dr. Isaac Golden, PhD, DHom, ND.
5. **Vaccination & Homoeoprophylaxis? - A Review of Risks and Alternatives**. (7th Ed.). Dr. Isaac Golden, PhD, DHom, ND.
6. **Homoeoprophylaxis - A Fifteen Year Clinical Study**. A Statistical Review of the Efficacy and Safety of Long-Term Homoeoprophylaxis. Dr. Isaac Golden PhD, DHom, ND.
7. **Vaccines 2.0**. The Careful Parent's Guide to Making Safe Vaccination Choices for Your Family. Mark Blaxill and Dan Olmsted.
8. **Immunisation Options: A Simple Guide for Parents Who Care**. Dr. Isaac Golden, PhD, DHom, ND.
9. **Vaccination is Not Immunization: The War On Children.** Tim O'Shea.

Acknowledgments

To understand the work presented here we must acknowledge that it would not be possible without the foundation of homeopathy and its propagation throughout the world. It is with deep respect and gratitude we thank Dr. Samuel Hahnemann for the genius of homeopathy and its applications in infectious disease prevention and treatment.

It is with much appreciation we acknowledge the pioneering work of Dr. Isaac Golden in homeoprophylaxis (HP) for childhood diseases, and his dedication to our process in analysis and preparation of the research for these publications. It was his work from 1985-2010 that provided the inspiration, underpinnings, and completion for the research presented here. Thank you to Dr. Gustov Bracho, with whom Kate Birch met a number of times following her first visit to Cuba. On each meeting, their heart-felt connections continued to grow as they shared a similar desire to truly help humanity and gratitude towards homeopathy for enabling this vision to unfold.

Thank you to Cilla Whatcott who partnered with Kate Birch in the writing of The Solution as they set forth the task of educating the public on homeoprophylaxis. Without the consumer demand for an alternative to vaccination, and a method of disease prevention that did not harm their children, there would be no path for the advancement of homeoprophylaxis. We are grateful to know that their work answered an emerging call from concerned families. Thank you to those families that invested in HP, the research and continued their relationship with Free and Healthy Children International (FHCi). You have been a forerunner for other families looking to make choices about how to educate their children's immune systems.

Thank you to the founding FHCi Board Members who championed this same vision of creating an avenue of access to HP in North America: Kate Birch, Cilla Whatcott, Rachel Kimbrel, Mila Krol, and Dr. Kim Lane who continued to be the medical advisor with FHCi through the publication of the research. Thank you to the HP Supervisors who implemented the research registration into their practices. Thank you to all those who helped in the compilation, analysis, and publication of the data: Kate Birch for the foresight and fortitude for maintaining the vision through to completion; Su Sandon for her impeccable diligence to ten years of tireless data entry; Katie Bromme and Max Sagert for the love, humor, and profound personal revelations they tapped into during data analysis process in 2019; and Sarah Damlo for her patient expertise in editing, proofreading, and administrative efforts towards tracking documents and verification of results.

Thank you to all past and current FHCi Board Members who have been with FHCi since founding in 2011. Most especially, to the four new HP Family Members, who invested the health of their own children in HP, and from their personal experience, joined the board in 2020 to work towards amplifying our vision into the public eye.

Thank you to our patrons for your generous donations throughout the last ten years to support completion of this research.

We are all part of a growing movement of understanding how the immune system works and how homeoprophylaxis can facilitate the healthy maturation of children. We are all vested in providing parental choice concerning what medicine to choose, which serves, not only the healthy immune development of their children, but also public health.

Lastly and most importantly, thank you to the children who have shown us how their immune systems work and how they work in response to HP. Without you, our research is nothing. Because of your positive and beneficial responses, we would not have an avenue of hope.

Thank you all for delivering free and healthy children to humanity!

Preface

There is a growing body of evidence that childhood vaccination programs are unduly burdening the health of children and subsequently future generations. The call the work of homeoprophylaxis was based the exponential increase of allergies, skin conditions, neurological and development disorders, learning and behavioral disorders, ADD, ADHD, and autism in children since the inception of the National Childhood Vaccine Injury Act of 1986 was

Since the mid 1990's, as a homeopath I asked what can be done to help change this trajectory. Circumstance took me to travel around the world while I was looking for answers to this problem. In 2008, I was invited to Cuba to present at a conference on the use of nosodes for large scale interventions in infectious disease with homeoprophylaxis. This prompted the development of Free and Healthy Children International (FHCi) to carry out research in homeoprophylaxis (HP) in North America. Now that the work is published, our duty is to bring public awareness to HP.

FHCi is a 501(c)3 dedicated to research, education, and access for the community to homeoprophylaxis. In 2009, we embarked on a ten-year research project which included educating practitioners and the public about HP and the supervision of children, aged newborn to 10 years, though our HP program. Part One of the research was published in December of 2019 and Part Two in June of 2020. Since the close of the research entrance in 2014, FHCi has continued to provide access to HP through our HP Family Membership platform. The year 2020 has been slated for public outreach to amplify our network and provide data for families to share within their communities explaining why they opted for HP over vaccines. This volume has been prepared for this task.

Interestingly, many of the families who registered for HP under the research had already completed the current vaccine schedule. Demonstrating that they either did not think the vaccines worked or they were hoping that HP would help overcome the deficits vaccination has left in their children. As we separated out the *Unvaccinated* from *Previously Vaccinated* cohorts, in the comparison of long-term health outcomes, we realized we had inadvertently also completed a vax/no-vax study in children. The results of these findings are tabulated throughout this publication.

The primary goal of providing a compilation of our research in one volume is to provide a tangible document which can be used to influence our community, doctors, and political leaders. Right now, we are living in a critical time in history where political powers have convinced us vaccines are the only way to prevent disease, and they are working on legislative measures that mandate allopathic methods. This dogma believes vaccines are the be-all-and-end-all methodology for disease prevention. However, many individuals and families are working to find holistic methods to maintain a healthy immune system in the face of infectious disease. HP answers this call. If we can discuss this option in an educated way, and have research to back up the conversation with our legislators, then we might have a tool by which we can work towards maintaining our rights to choose the medical procedures we desire for ourselves and our children. It is for these reasons we present this work.

Know our effort is for the betterment of humanity, for the health of children, and to support the rational implementation of a homeopathic public health model that originates from a place of benevolence towards understanding the fragility of humanity and the beneficial and pathological effects of the bacterial and viral environments we have co-evolved in.

I am honored to be the one called to present this here.

In service,

Kate Birch RSHom, RSHom(NA), CCH. July 27, 2020

Forward

There are 4 main sections in this book:

    a. Introduction.

This is an overview of the philosophical orientation to the work of homeopathy and homeoprophylaxis. At the outset, as we have delineated some results between the *Unvaccinated* and *Previously Vaccinated* cohorts, there is a review and discussion on the differences between the methodology of HP compared to Vaccination.

Here, we also differentiate types of research and whether or not our research confirms the philosophical understanding of homeopathy, HP, and infectious disease. As the research papers and initial article do not expressly explain the process, vocabulary definitions, or theoretical understanding of HP, the introduction serves to present the topic, and background that went into the study, and also serves as a template upon which to comprehend the results. Commentary and criticism of the research is also reviewed in this section. As a result of our findings, FHCi implemented a number of changes and improvements to the program and delivery/supervision to enhance compliance and health outcomes. These additions and changes are also discussed here.

The following three articles are published in their entirety without edits or commentary. Each article remains in their original published form. As these articles were published at different times in different journals, you will find duplication of some of the material. Please also refer to the Index of Tables to navigate the data. The unique numeric identification of each table is maintained through each article. For example, the tables that are from Part One are numbered 1.1, 1.2 etc. Tables numbered 2.1, 2.2 etc. are from Part Two. Accordingly, Table 2.1.a. from the American Homeopath is referenced from Part Two of the long-term research publication. The introduction is followed by a short Glossary of Terms.

    b. One journal article, Establishing Homeoprophylaxis as a Public Health Care Model, overviews the history and the vision of the application of HP in North America.*

    c. Two peer reviewed research articles published based on the effectiveness of Homeoprophylaxis*** in Children in North America in Similia; The Journal of the Australian Society of Homeopaths.*****

The articles published in Australia use British English in content and the 'oeo' diphthong in Homoeopathy and Homoeoprophylaxis. Accordingly, you will see this spelling and grammatical usage throughout.

    d. Appendix of supplemental tables not included in the published articles.

Not all tables were included in the publication of Part Two thus justifying the need for this volume to expound and provide more background data for the summaries and conclusions. These tables are numerated 3.2.1, 3.2.2, etc. denoting that they are a continuation of the themes summarized in Part Two. The additional digits link them to their respective themes. I.e. Table 2.3.1. Unique symptoms elicited from Pertussin is the third theme in Part Two and Table 3.2.3.1.a. Unique and common symptoms in response to Pertussin, is the comprehensive listing of symptoms in the Appendix. In the Appendix is Table 3.3 summarizes the number of children exposed to indicated diseases as compared to contraction rates. This table is not in the published results because the numbers of those exposed compared to those who contracted was too small to give any significant numbers of efficacy of HP. That said we included the table here to demonstrate that there is more work needed in this area of research.****

As FHCi is dedicated to research, we have established a platform for continued work on other disease outbreaks. Currently, humanity is preoccupied with Coronavirus. This is an exciting time to be alive and to be participating in the evolution of public health programs. Accordingly, FHCi has embarked on research on the use of Novus-CV nosode for prevention and treatment. Please look for the publication of this work in the Fall of 2020.

* North America: FHCi oversees HP Supervisors administering the program in Canada and the United States. All participants in both countries follow the same procedures, consent and follow up forms, and have full access to the supervision built within the program.

** Effectiveness Vs Efficacy: Effective treatment provides positive results in a usual or routine care condition that may or may not be controlled for research purposes but may be controlled in the sense that specific activities are undertaken to increase the likelihood of positive results. Effectiveness studies use real-world clinicians and clients, and clients who have multiple diagnoses or needs. In this case effectiveness would mean that despite exposure to an infectious illness the disease was not contracted alongside qualitative health outcome measures. In contrast, Efficacious treatment (Efficacy) provides positive results in a controlled experimental research trial. A study that shows a treatment approach to be "efficacious" means that the study produced good outcomes which were identified in advance, in a controlled experimental trial, often in highly constrained conditions, double blinded and randomized. Efficacy may mean the ability to produce antibody titers as a quantitative analysis.

***Homeoprophylaxis (HP): the use of highly diluted and succussed (potentized) substances given by oral ingestion prior to exposure to disease with the aim to prevent that disease. These medicinal agents are made from matter either in the natural world: plant, mineral, or animal extracts, e.g. homeopathic remedies: cultured pathogens, and/or human discharges produced in response to those pathogens, e.g. nosodes as per outlined in the HPUS (Homeopathic Pharmacopeia of the United States, FDA regulated).

**** Ethics in research demands protecting the autonomy of the individual research subject, insisting on informed consent and a reasonable risk/benefit ratio for a study to be ethical. In research, the risks to participants must be considered in assessing the risk/benefit ratio of study designs. For all research regarding efficacy towards the prevention of infectious disease it is considered unethical to directly expose individuals to infectious disease to determine if a prevention is effective. For this reason, we have not directly exposed participants to infectious diseases and can only rely on random exposure relative to infectious disease rates in the public to evaluate efficacy of HP. Accordingly, our research does not specifically address the efficacy of HP towards infectious disease prevention. Rather, our research looks at the level of compliance to the completion of the HP program (Part One) and the immediate and long-term health effects of HP (Part Two). For these reasons we also call HP an immune system education process rather than a disease prevention method. This is based on the understanding that healthy immune systems know how to process childhood infectious diseases. Our research demonstrates positive effects of HP towards strengthening children's overall health.

Table of Contents

Acknowledgments...i

Preface...iii

Forward...v

Index of Tables..ix

Introduction 1

Glossary of Terms 15

1. Establishing Homeoprophylaxis as a Public Healthcare Model...17

2. Long-term homoeoprophylaxis study in children in North America. Part One: Factors contributing to the successful completion of sequential dosing of disease nosodes.*.................................29

    Abstract...29

    Introduction 30

    Research Question 30

    Method...30

    Parameters of Research 31

    Results...35

    Discussion 45

    Conclusions...47

    Economic disclosure 48

    References* 49

3. Long-term homoeoprophylaxis study in children in North America. Part Two: Safety of HP, review of immunological responses, and effects on general health outcomes...51

    Abstract...51

    Introduction 52

    Research Questions 53

    Method...53

    Parameters of Research 53

    Results...57

    Discussion 70

    Conclusions...71

    Economic disclosure 72

    References* 73

4. Appendix 75

Index of Tables

Chart 1. Nosodes for a general disease prevention protocol 6

Chart A. Homoeoprophylaxis program (Prophylaxis Record) 34, 56

Chart B. Homeoprophylaxis program 2019 (Prophylaxis record) 10

Figure 1. Circle of natural disease 7

Figure 2. Primary and secondary action of drugs 8

Figure 3. Number of children doing HP with FHCi 2009-2019 12

Figure 4. Bell curve of infectious disease over time in the general population 18

Figure 5. Research with antibody production in mice with nosoLEP 19

Figure 6. Economic disclosure for Part One and Two 26

Figure 7. Inclusion/Exclusion criteria 31

Table 1.1.a. Total number, gender, and previous vaccination status of registrants at all levels of completion 22

Table 1.1.b. Total number of registrants and levels of completion
Comparing girls and boys 35

Table 1.1.c. Totals of *Unvaccinated* and *Previously Vaccinated* at all levels of completion 57

Table 1.2. Age groups of registrants 36

Table 1.3. CDC early childhood immunisation schedule 37

Table 1.4. Total number of previous vaccine-disease doses per child at registration and at various stages of the program 38

Table 1.5.a. -1.5.g.
Socio-economic data of registrants in values and percentages 42

Table 1.6. Reasons for Withdrew or Starting and Stopping 43

Table 1.7. Comparison of regional distribution of HP Supervisors and children at registration and upon completion of document tracking 44

Table 2.1.a. Total number of nosode/remedy responses as compared to dosing series recorded 23, 58

Table 2.1.b. Adverse events reported 23, 58

Table 2.1.c. Total number of *Unvaccinated* and *Previously Vaccinated* respondents with documented symptoms per nosode/remedy 59

Table 2.1.d. Total number of responses to nosodes/remedies for the entire program 60

Table 2.1.e. Total number of responses per dosing series 60

Table 2.1.f. Total # of responses recorded and # individual doses as compared to # of dosing series given 62

Table 2.2. Comparing frequency of incidence in general health outcomes of *Unvaccinated* and *Previously Vaccinated* to national incidence in those *Completed* 25

Table 2.2.a. General health outcomes of *Unvaccinated* and *Previously Vaccinated* in *Completed in 50 months* compared to National incidence 63

Table 2.2.b. Comparison of Initial and Final Health Profiles of *Unvaccinated* and *Previously Vaccinated* who *Completed* in 50 months 65

Table 2.2.c. Comparison of Initial and Final Health Profiles 66

Table 2.3. "Common symptom" nosode/remedy responses 67

Table 2.3.1. Unique symptoms elicited from Pertussin 67

Table 2.3.2. Unique symptoms elicited from Pneumococcinum 68

Table 2.3.3. Unique symptoms elicited from Lathyrus sativus 68

Table 2.3.4. Unique symptoms elicited from Haemophilus 68

Table 2.3.5. Unique symptoms elicited from Meningococcinum 69

Table 2.3.6. Unique symptoms elicited from Tetanus toxin 69

Table 2.3.7. Unique symptoms elicited from Parotidinum 69

Table 2.3.8. Unique symptoms elicited from Morbillinum 69

Table 3.2.1.a a. Number of children with recorded number of responses from each dosing series 76

Table 3.2.2.d. Health Profiles of *Unvaccinated* who *Completed* upon registration and at the end of the program. 77

Table 3.2.2.e. Frequency of Conditions in all *Unvaccinated* at all four stages of the program 79

Table 3.2.2.f. Health Profiles of *Previously Vaccinated* who *Completed* upon registration and at the end of the program 80

Table 3.2.2.g. Health profiles of all *Previously Vaccinated* at all four stages of the program 82

Table 3.2.3.1.a. Unique and common symptoms in response to Pertussin 84

Table 3.2.3.2.a. Unique and common symptoms in response to Pneumococcinum 84

Table 3.2.3.3.a. Unique and common symptoms in response to Lathyrus sativus 84

Table 3.2.3.4.a. Unique and common symptoms in response to Haemophilus influenzae 85

Table 3.2.3.6.a. Unique and common symptoms in response to Tetanus toxin 86

Table 3.2.3.8.a. Unique and common symptoms in response to Morbillinum 87

Table 3.2.4. Number of children exposed to disease versus contraction rates 88

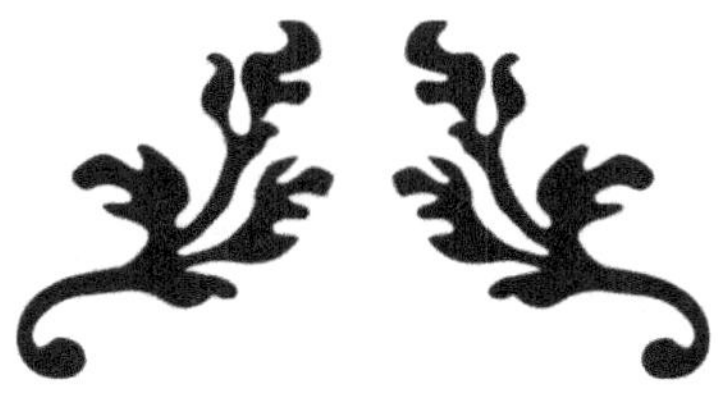

In reference to the healing potential
of disease matter -

Whether derived from the purist gold
or the purist filth our gratitude for its
excellence in service forbids us to
inquire or care.

P.B. Bell

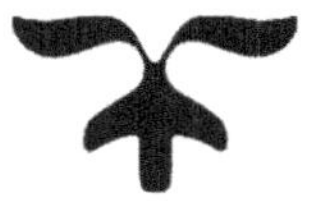

Introduction

Comparison of Homeopathy and Homeoprophylaxis

Before embarking on presenting and interpreting the results of this homeoprophylaxis (HP) research we must first compare and contrast the basic principles of homeopathy and HP. While homeopathy is a complete system into itself, homeoprophylaxis is described by both comparable and opposing philosophical constructs. Both are comprehensive systems of medicine backed by understanding that the true nature of the cause of disease and the subsequent ability for the body to contract and heal from infectious disease is an internal mechanism (susceptibility) in relation to the virility of the disease. This applies to acute infectious disease and also chronic disease. While homeopathy is based on the 'Law of Similars' (similar disease) as the mechanism of cure, by reducing susceptibility, there is debate whether HP is acting on this curative principle or the principle of 'dissimilar disease' (as described below). The following is an overview of the founding principles of HP and reflections on mode of action.

While the popular view of acute disease is that it should be avoided at all costs, and the current use of vaccination is to these ends, we have forgotten the positive role acute disease can play in childhood development and the need for a healthy immune system to process that disease. To be clear on this point, this research is not about how to use HP to stop acute infectious disease. But rather, it is to overview how the systematic use of homeopathic nosodes lessens susceptibility to infectious disease, strengthens the immune system, and reduces the need for acute disease. Because HP activates an immunological response relative to a disease agent, in doing so, HP reduces susceptibility to contract the disease.

> While a nosode has the ability to produce an immune system response, the extent to which the body reacts is not as extreme as it would be if acted upon by the actual germ, because we can adjust the potency and frequency of repetition according to the person's sensitivity. Thus nosodes, when administered in the appropriate dose, act to tone an individual's health in a controlled manner.

Comparison of Homeoprophylaxis and Vaccination

Historically, with the smallpox epidemics in Europe, it was observed that those who previously contracted cowpox were immune to smallpox. This observation led scientists to the idea of inoculating people with cowpox disease to prevent smallpox. This was the first instance of vaccination used in people. The cowpox material inoculated under the skin produced a mild local eruptive response (termed Vaccinia) similar to that of smallpox and, in some people, generated life-long immunity to smallpox. At this same time homeopaths developed a homeopathic preparation (dilution) from a smallpox vesicle and used this with equal effectiveness for the prevention of smallpox. This homeopathic nosode was called Variolinum.

Contemporaries to the Jenner smallpox vaccine researched the potential of preventing other diseases by introducing live viruses to stimulate immunity. Experiments were begun with dogs and the rabies virus. Unfortunately, this method killed many dogs until Louis Pasteur had the idea to incubate the virus in rabbits to lessen its virulence. This was the first attempt at attenuation, the weakening of the virulence of a disease.

This method of attenuating the virus in another host species tissue is still used today in the production of vaccines. Homeopathic attenuation is achieved through dilution and succession of the original discharge.

Issues with the vaccine method are four-fold:

1. The final product not only has the original pathogen but also the possibility of pathogens found in the host cell culture,[i; ii] viruses, and also, DNA from the host cells. Inoculation of this genetic material can import undesirable effects in the recipient's DNA.
2. Vaccines are stabilized with a variety of other ingredients such as bovine casein, peanut oil, antibiotics, yeast, and also aluminum adjuvants, which force the immune system into a hyperactive allergic response to not only the infectious agent but also the other ingredients. In many vaccines the mercury containing preservative Thimerosal is used.
3. Vaccines are injected into muscle tissue, subsequently bypassing the peripheral aspects of the immune system, which are on the mucous membranes. Importing infectious agents directly into the body leads to confusion for the specific elimination pathway that disease needs.
4. The CDC vaccine schedule in use now calls for multiple disease agents to be administered simultaneously and frequently over a short amount of time. Infants' immune systems are too immature to develop the appropriate immunological response to so many diseases at once and recover in time for the subsequent doses.

As a result of the vaccination method, the ill-health of children in America has reached epidemic proportions.[iii,iv,v, vi] It is for these reasons we need Homeoprophylaxis (HP). It is a time-honored practice of infectious disease prevention and its effectiveness is well-documented throughout history for the last 200 years.[vii,viii]

The main differences between homeoprophylaxis and vaccination is the method of attenuation, delivery, and dosing schedule.

Similarities between HP and Vaccination:
- Aim to prevent disease
- Derived from actual disease
- Aim to stimulate immunity prior to exposure of infectious disease

Differences:

Homeoprophylaxis:
- Uses a single disease at a time
- Targets general immune system to function and respond appropriately
- Given by mouth
- Attenuation by dilution
- Has no chemicals or additives

Vaccination:
- Administers multiple diseases at once
- Targets specific antibody production expectation (not possible till 12-24 months of age)
- Injected into muscle
- Includes toxins, crude bacterial or viral doses, and human and non-human DNA
- Has added chemicals: preservatives, mercury, adjuvants, aluminum, and antibiotics

Outcomes:
- Homeoprophylaxis offers mild immunological responses which serve to educate the immune system resulting in immune system integrity.
- Vaccination results in many potential side effects including eczema, encephalitis, auto-immune conditions and even death, as a result of too many diseases given at once resulting in immune system confusion.

                                        Introduction

What is Homeopathy?

German physician Samuel Hahnemann developed the system of homeopathy at the turn of the eighteenth century. Hahnemann lived when epidemics still ravaged most of Europe. At that time, the diseases of rabies, smallpox, influenza, diphtheria, tuberculosis, scarlet fever, syphilis, gonorrhea, etc. were common in most populations. The concept of contagion was still a mystery. Superstitious and underdeveloped theories dominated the medical practice of the day. Bacteria and viruses had not yet been identified. In fact, the "Germ Theory" as developed by Louis Pasteur, Robert Koch, and contemporary scientific researchers, was not presented until after Hahnemann died. Herbology was in its rudiments and heroic medical practices such as bloodletting, strong dosing with mercurial medicaments, and leeches, were considered the norm. Basic anatomy was still a frontier science. None-the-less, Hahnemann identified the basic principles of infectious disease and initiated public health measures to treat and prevent epidemics during his time. He worked with scarlet fever, rabies, Asiatic cholera, typhus, and others.

Law of Similars

It was during this time that not only did he become well educated in the scientific realm he also began to speculate upon the nature of cure and to develop a system of healing that would result in permanent resolution. Through his studies, he came upon the concept of "like treats like."

This concept reasoned that a medicament could treat a disease because
it had the power to cause a similar disease.

He experimented to test this theory and developed a process called a "proving," whereby he ingested a substance and over the following hours, days, and weeks he meticulously recorded the nature of symptoms he developed. Hahnemann documented these symptoms and catalogued them in his Materia Medica (catalogue of remedies and their symptomatology). This Materia Medica is still in use today and the same remedies that were used for fevers or vomiting and diarrhea then are in use today. The human response to disease has remained the same even if variants of the infectious agents have changed. I.e. Influenza activates fever, chill, and body aches regardless of the seasonal strain.

Theory and Method of HP

Nosodes are a specific category of remedies made from infectious disease or pathological discharge or tissue. The goal of taking a nosode is to produce an immunological response much like a proving does. Documentation of these symptoms provides indications for the homeopathic use of these nosodes (curative action).

Homeoprophylaxis satisfies the process of naturally acquired disease by providing a tiny dose of the disease, but without any of the risks.

Nosodes are given orally, one disease at a time and work to stimulate general immunity. The immunity engendered is much like the immunity of naturally acquired disease. HP is administered to children through the sequential dosing of specific nosodes, in various potencies, over several months or years during which their immune systems are developing. This dosing schedule activates mild normal disease-specific immune responses, as if they have encountered the disease.

The attenuation process used in the preparation of a nosode dilutes out any disease material so one does not contract the disease, nor do any of the immune responses developed in relation to the nosode render the pathogen to be contagious from one child to another. The stimulated response symptoms pass away as an adaptation process of developing immunity. It is this process that lowers susceptibility to contraction of disease and builds the flexibility of the immune system to function optimally in relation to the environment and other infectious agents while supporting the normal stages of childhood development.

The precept is that childhood infectious diseases are intended to
be contracted in childhood: the immunological processes
stimulated by these diseases help to mature the child's immune
system. HP serves to activate immune responses without putting
the child at risk of the actual disease.

Homeopathic (Similar) Diseases

In *The Organon of Medicine*,[ix] Hahnemann demonstrates that not only is it possible that a contagion with a specific disease expression can set up a state of chronic ill-health, or miasm, but that these same diseases can also be homeopathic (similar in symptoms expression) and therefore curative to an existing latent miasm of the child or person.[x] A latent miasm is a preexisting condition set up from incomplete resolution of a previously contracted disease process, passed down from generation to generation, that when sufficiently stimulated by adverse conditions, may be activated to develop chronic disease in the offspring. The immune system processes generated by childhood infectious disease are intended to release the child from the burden (miasm) of a latent miasm and inherited weaknesses.

The Law of Similars is a universal law. Any agent that has the ability to make an effect has the same ability to ameliorate that effect. Correspondingly, it is possible that an infectious disease has the potential to be curative to a similar underlying susceptibility.

Hahnemann postulated further that rather than exposing oneself
to the crude disease to obtain immunity, why not administer a
homeopathic preparation of the disease to engender immunity.
This is what nosodes are for.

Dissimilar diseases

In the *Organon of Medicine,* in paragraphs 34-40, Hahnemann describes the principles of dissimilar disease as opposed to similar diseases to which the rest of the *Organon* is devoted.[xi] The aphorisms propose that the body has three possible responses.

1. If the strength of the existing state of health is stronger than the new disease, the new disease is not therefore contracted and thus *repelled.*
2. If the strength of the new disease is stronger than that of the pre-existing disease of the individual, the original state of health is *suspended* while the immune system processes and resolves the new disease.
3. If the strength of the original state of health is neither weaker nor stronger than the new disease, the vital force can neither repel nor resolve the disease. The result is a *complex disease* whereby the new disease settles into its organ of affinity and renders the individual in a state of never well since which will carry on in its trajectory unless treated by medicine.

Origins of Homeoprophylaxis

James Compton Burnett, a homeopath contemporary to the development of the smallpox and rabies vaccines in the 1800's, was the first doctor to forcefully warn against the dangers of vaccination and the use of material disease agents to protect against serious diseases. He believed that vaccination generated a state of disease of its own resulting in its own latent miasm.

He postulated that if the appropriate immune system reaction was not developed, the effect was for the injected pathogenic material to pollute the body and result in a state of chronic disease he called **vaccinosis**. This is the complex disease option number three as mentioned above.

Burnett argued that vaccination, as practiced by Edward Jenner or Louis Pasteur, using material doses of cowpox or rabies (the first diseases vaccines were created with cowpox for smallpox and rabies respectively), would eventually end in disaster because it was only temporary protection. It did not individualize the dose to the health of the individual and would ultimately cause long-term chronic consequences.

> Burnett proposed the use of a homeopathic potency of the disease as a less harmful way to encourage an immune system response without the introduction of the actual disease material into the blood.

The use of homeopathic nosode, *Variolinum* (the nosode derived from smallpox pustule) introduced into homeopathic practice was an early instance of HP. Disease specific remedies in the homeopathic Materia Medica could also be used for HP.

HP was previously documented in 1801 when Samuel Hahnemann described using *Belladonna* for the prevention of scarlet fever.[xii] Since that time, homeopathy has treated and homeoprophylaxis has successfully prevented a variety of illnesses, including childhood diseases, as well as serious epidemics and tropical diseases.

Homeopathic Attenuation by Dilution

To "attenuate" means to make something smaller or weaker. In electronics, reducing the amplification of a signal without distorting its sound is known as attenuation. A fever can be attenuated, or reduced, by cool bathing. A virus or bacteria can be attenuated by a variety of methods. Homeopathic nosodes, are attenuated through a careful process called "potentization." Vaccine materials are attenuated (weakened virility) by denaturing, radiation, incubation in a foreign host medium, or other methods.

Potentization is a method by which the original pathogen is passed through a series of repeated dilutions. Each dilution is followed by "succussion," or the forceful striking of the vessel containing the solution against a hard surface. With the pathogen diluted to the point of no original molecules, and having been succussed, only its energetic frequency remains in solution.[xiii] It is no longer virulent or dangerous in any way.

All material, biological and otherwise, possesses a unique energetic signature, or frequency. Diluted preparations of disease agents have been shown to emit the same energetic frequency as the original disease agent.[xiv] This frequency is sufficient to stimulate general immune system function.

Because all homeopathic remedies are potentized, the original culture or specimen can be infinitely reproduced from one original source.

Nosodes are made without additives, adjuvants (chemicals intended to increase the action of vaccines), or preservatives. Nor are they incubated on any animal or human fetal tissue. Nosodes are administered orally and one at a time. By touching upon the mucus membranes of the mouth, the body's first line of defense, they stimulate the normal order of eliminatory immune system processes.

The homeopathic nosodes used in the FHCi HP program are derived from the discharges of active and serologically confirmed disease expression in children in San Diego Hospital (CA) from 2000-2009.[xv]

Sources of Nosodes

- Sputum or nasal discharges
- Scrapings from mucous membranes, vesicles or cankers, pathological tissue such as cancerous tumors or tubercular encasements
- Pathological blood
- Decomposed matter
- Cultured bacteria, viruses, or vaccines
- Examples below

• ***Diphtherinum*** - Diphtheria	• ***Pertussin*** - Whooping cough
• ***Haemophilus influenzinum*** - Haemophilus Influenzae B	• ***Pneumococcinum*** - Pneumococcal disease
• ***Hepatitis A nosode, Hepatitis B nosode*** - Hepatitis A or B	• ***Polio nosode*** - Poliomyelitis
• ***Human papilloma virus nosode*** - HPV. Not in Study	• ***Rotavirus nosode*** - Rotavirus. Not in Study
• ***Influenzinum*** - Influenza. Not in Study	• ***Rubella nosode*** - German measles. Not in Study
• ***Meningococcinum*** - Meningococcal disease	• ***Tetanus toxin*** - Tetanus toxin
• ***Morbillinum*** - Measles	• ***Varicella*** - Chickenpox
• ***Parotidinum*** - Mumps	

Chart 1. Nosodes for a general disease prevention protocol

Healthy Immune Response

In order to have a healthy immune system, the immune system must know how to develop a fever and resolve that fever. Immunity develops through a subtle interaction between disease agents and the innate intelligence of the body.

The system of homeopathy has both remedies and nosodes that facilitate this process. These are selected homeopathically by their symptom specificity to the symptoms presenting in the patient. An HP nosode will activate the immune system process that acute disease needs to resolve itself. Nosodes can be used before, during, and after contraction of infectious disease.

- When a nosode is used *before* exposure to disease this is homeoprophylaxis. When given before exposure and symptoms develop this immune system process mimics the natural disease process and relinquishes the need of the disease to do the same.
- When used *during* active disease this action is supportive to the immune process intended to resolve the disease and will provide stimulus to move the individual through that process.
- When used *after* an active acute disease, in cases sequalae since infectious disease, a nosode acts curatively.

Introduction

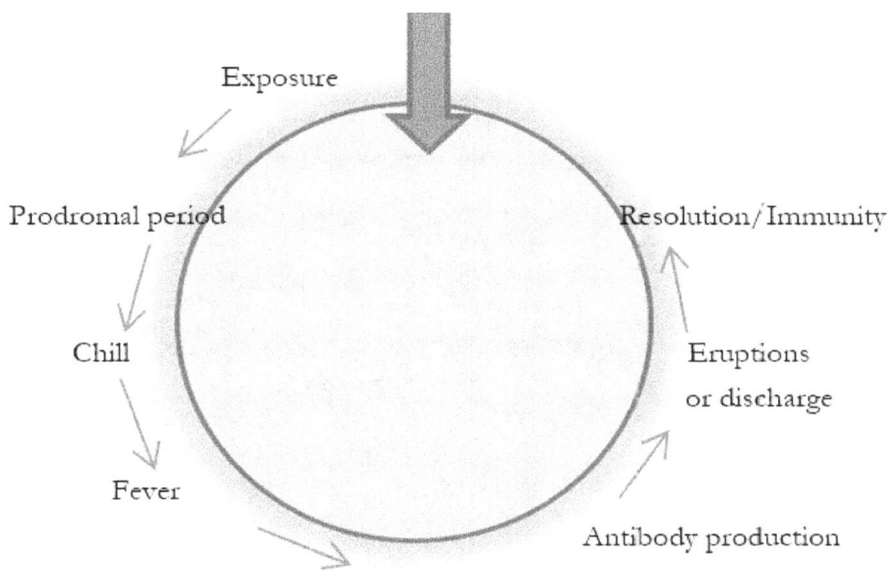

Figure 1. Circle of natural disease

Primary and Secondary Action of Drugs

Every medicinal substance has a primary action and a secondary action. The primary action is what the substance does to the person. The secondary action is what the vital force of the body does in response to the substance. In material doses (substances in crude form) the secondary action to a substance is usually in equal and opposite force to the primary action. Such as, if you consume a poison the body will violently purge itself to overcome the primary poisoning action. Most allopathic drugs rely upon the primary action and what it does to the body to control symptoms. The side-effects are the fall out of the body's response to this drug (secondary action).

The process of potentization for homeopathic remedies reduces a substance's primary action, while increasing the potential of the secondary action *if* the substance is homeopathic in its indications to the ailments of the person. For example, if you are hyper of mind and can't sleep, the remedy **Coffea**, (which corresponds to those symptoms) can facilitate the body to rebalance that disturbance.

The general concept of homeopathy is to activate the secondary action of the human response to sickness or stress which brings about healing. The following diagrams depict this action in comparison to allopathic drugs. In HP there are two possible scenarios of action. Either that of dissimilar disease whereby we rely upon the primary action of the HP nosode to activate an immune response of the individual. *Or*, the primary action of the nosode activates a secondary action which is curative to the pre-existing susceptibility. The rest time between subsequent doses allows for an adaptive process of the immune system to reconcile the information presented from exposure to the diluted preparation of the disease agent. This adaptive response may be a curative response, as in a lessening of susceptibility to infectious disease, or simply a bi-phasal action/reaction process that results in immunity.

This diagram below depicts this concept:

1. Allopathic meds work on <u>primary action</u> of the drug to suppress symptoms. <u>The secondary action</u> is that of the vital force responding back to the drug.

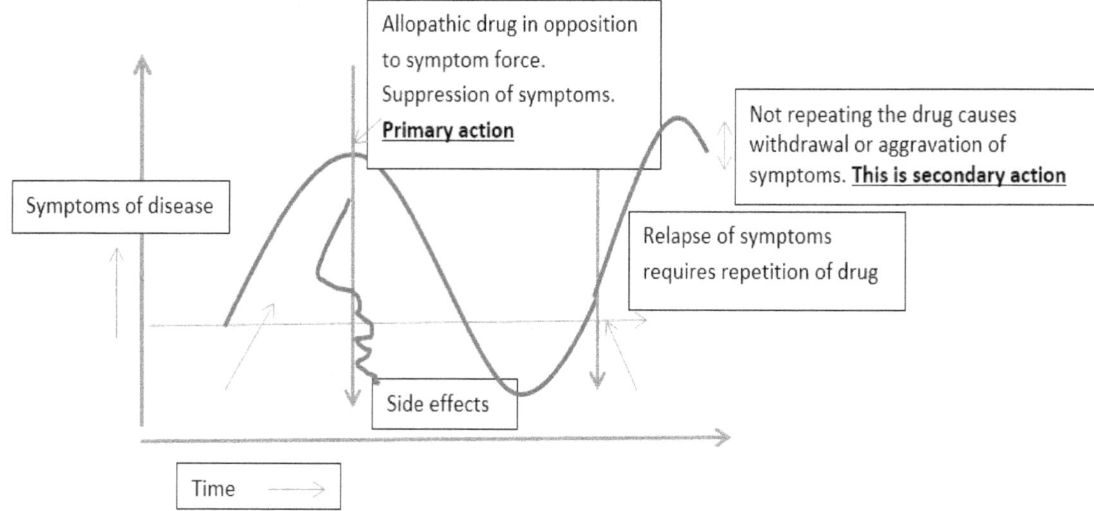

2. Homeopathic remedies work to awaken **secondary action**. **The primary action** is along the same lines of the person's symptoms then the secondary response is for the body to not produce these symptoms.

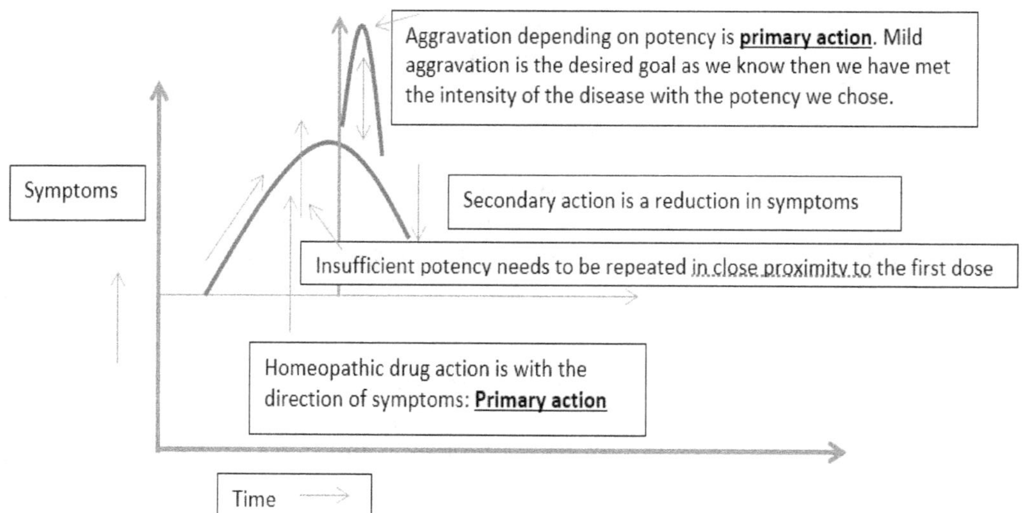

Figure 2. Primary and secondary action of drugs

Commentary on Research Findings

This was a real-time long-term effectiveness study in children from multiple socio-economic backgrounds and varied immunological status prior to entry into the program. We were looking to answer two main questions:

1. Can parents complete a self-administered immune system education program with homeopathic nosodes of infectious disease agents with their children?
2. How does the application of sequential dosing of infectious disease nosodes affect children's health, and what are the effects of nosodes in participants?

While this research is not finite, and there were many confounders, we do have some statistically significant results demonstrating the beneficial outcomes of HP in children's health.

> This research was not designed to prove that homeopathy works nor if
> HP is effective for disease prevention. It is to determine *if* there were
> effects of nosodes on immune health and *what* were those effects?

Results

- This research demonstrates that there are unique immunological responses with individual nosodes in children, and these responses appeared to enhance their health.
- These effects are in line with the philosophy of homeoprophylaxis and serve to validify the use of HP for healthy immune system development.
- This alone demonstrates that homeoprophylaxis has the potential to be vital to the global health care crisis with regards to infectious disease and children's health.

That said, there were a number of research design flaws which led to insufficient data collection but also inspired important changes and updates to the program FHCi offers:

Health Intake and Registration

- We falsely started from the assumption that all children coming to HP had a healthy immune system foundation.
- A number of registrant children had pre-existing medical conditions affecting healthy immune system responses to the nosodes.
- We were naive to the effects of antibiotics in the mothers' health history, pregnancy, and birth process on infants' immune system function.
- We had incomplete inclusion/exclusion criteria
    - With regards to the mother's health and birth of the child.
    - Previous use of medications or antibiotics in the mother and child.
- We underestimated the lack of education in the general public about healthy immune system function and the potential environmental and lifestyle confounders to healthy immune system function.

- FHCi implemented a more comprehensive intake form and recommends constitutional homeopathic care to clear the effects of antibiotics, vaccinations and/or medications given to the mother in pregnancy or during childbirth.
- We developed teaching materials to support natural childbirth, organic foods sources, and the benefits of breast milk over formula.
- We changed the order of remedies in the program to include **Polio** rather than **Lathyrus sativus** (which historically was used to treat and prevent Polio). Previous research shows that Polio virus (as in wild or the oral polio vaccine given in infancy) supports healthy intestinal and subsequent immune system function by closing the tight junctions of the intestinal wall. [xvi] Appropriately gapped tight junctions support healthy digestion and immune system function. **Polio** nosode serves to facilitate this process without the risk of the actual disease.[xvii]
- We now introduce **Polio** as the first remedy in the beginning of the program to address this issue.
- We added **Streptococcinum** to the program as "streptococcal infection" is the primary reason parents will turn to the use of antibiotics. Our understanding is that streptococcal bacteria are healthy commensal bacteria. It is only when the relationship to that bacteria is out of balance does the body fall ill and the fever produced in response is there to rebalance that relationship. By introducing **Streptococcinum** early in the program we are reducing the pathological streptococcal process AND limiting the introduction of yeast overgrowth and subsequent immune system changes that antibiotics bring about. Elevated Candida obscures healthy immune system function.
- **New program schedule:**

Monthly Doses	Remedy	Potency	Label	Date	Initials	Check for response, comment on notes pg. 25 -28
2 weeks	Polio	200	C1			
3 weeks	Polio	200 ,200, 200	C1			
5 weeks	Streptococcinum	200	S1			
6 weeks	Streptococcinum	200, 200, 200	S1			
2 months	Pertussin	200	A1			
3 months	Pertussin	200, 200, 200	A1			
4 months	Pneumococcinum	200	B1			
5 months	Pneumococcinum	200, 200, 200	B1			
6 months	Haemophilus (Hib)	200	D1			
7 months	Haemophilus (Hib)	200, 200, 200	D1			
8 months	Meningococcinum	200	E1			
9 months	Meningococcinum	200, 200, 200	E1			
10 months	Tetanus Toxin	200	F1			
11 months	Tetanus Toxin	200, 200, 200	F1			
12 months	Parotidinum	200	H1			
13 months	Parotidinum	200, 200, 200	H1			
14 months	Morbillinum	200	I1			
15 months	Morbillinum	200, 200, 200	I1			
16 months	Rest or Supplemental Program	See page 23				

Chart B Homeoprophylaxis program 2019 (Prophylaxis record)

Monthly	Remedy	Potency	Label	Date	Initials	Response
17 months	Polio	10M, 10M, 10M	C3			
18 months	Streptococcinum	10M, 10M, 10M	S3			
19 months	Pertussin	10M, 10M, 10M	A3			
20 months	Pneumococcinum	10M, 10M, 10M	B3			
21 months	Haemophilus (Hib)	10M, 10M, 10M	D3			
22 months	Meningococcinum	10M, 10M, 10M	E3			
23 months	Tetanus Toxin	10M, 10M, 10M	F3			
24 months	Parotidinum	10M, 10M, 10M	H3			
25 months	Morbillinum	10M, 10M, 10M	I3			
26 months	Supplemental Program	See Page 23				
Monthly	Remedy	Potency	Label	Date	Initials	Response
27 months	Polio	10M, 10M, 10M	C3			
29 months	Streptococcinum	10M, 10M, 10M	S3			
31 months	Pertussin	10M,10M, 10M	A3			
33 months	Pneumococcinum	10M, 10M, 10M	B3			
35 months	Haemophilus (Hib)	10M, 10M, 10M	D3			
37 months	Meningococcinum	10M, 10M, 10M	E3			
39 months	Tetanus Toxin	10M, 10M, 10M	F3			
41 months	Parotidinum	10M, 10M, 10M	H3			
43 months	Morbillinum	10M, 10M, 10M	I3			
45 months	Supplemental Program	See Page 23				

Remedy-Disease Relationship: Polio – Polio; Streptococcinum – Streptococcus; Pertussin - Whooping Cough; Pneumococcirum - Pneumococcus; Haemophilus -Haemophilus Influenzae Type B/Hib; Meningococcinum -Meningococcus; Tetanus Toxin - Tetanus; Parotidinum - Mumps; Morbillinum - Measles

Training of Practitioners

- We assumed HP Supervisors had sufficient education to discuss with perspective registrants how the program worked and when families were supposed to contact them for supervision.
    - o HP requires a paradigm shift of consumers and practitioners away from the concept of disease prevention towards education of the immune system. FHCi has implemented advanced trainings to further support our practitioners in their interface with families and the health of children undertaking HP.
- We underestimated the complexity of HP family's lives and their commitment to the process of HP, not only to give the doses according to the schedule, but to follow-up through the entire 44-month program.
    - o Through more extensive education of our HP Supervisors and through our HP Family Membership platform, we continue to encourage diligence to application of the program.
    - o Different schedules are being considered to more rapidly complete at least one series of diseases in the first year of the program.
    - o FHCi continues to explore educational platforms to help parents who choose HP not feel isolated in their communities and unsupported in their choice. This support is intended to give language to foster the HP paradigm.

Gleaning data

- We underestimated the multiplicity of confounding factors that set apart initial responses to HP remedies and long-term health outcomes.
    - While we have documented long-term health outcomes, some of the increased incidence of health conditions after HP may have to do with previous vaccinations, health choices of the parents, and environmental factors in differing geographical locations. For instance, those children who live in the Midwest with agricultural lands may have increased incidence of allergies due to pesticide exposure.
    - Closer examination of previous vaccination status would have more accurately clarified long-term health outcomes in the *Previously Vaccinated*.
    - With insufficient health history of mothers in pregnancy and childbirth, we do not know what, if any, factors contributed to the outcomes such as continuance with the program, remedy responses, and long-term outcomes.
- We underestimated the compliance needed of registrants and HP Supervisors to the document tracking process. The outcome of which weakened our research validity. However, while the numbers of respondents were small, we have confidence that the non-respondents had similar results to those documented.
    - We have since developed on-line documentation rather than paper for subsequent research designed to create more compliance and an increase in validity of research outcomes.

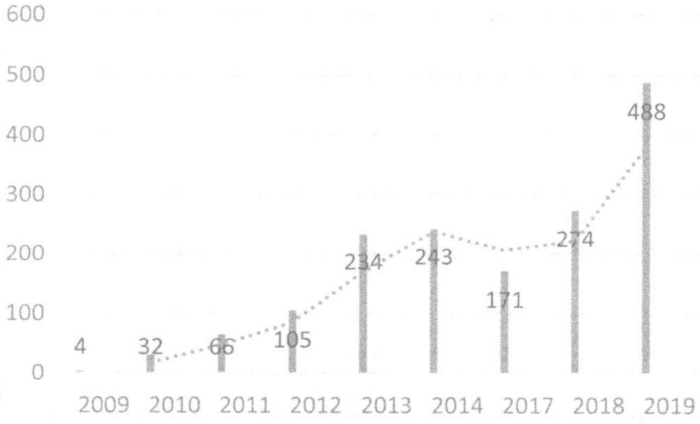

Figure 3. Number of children doing HP with FHCi: 2009-2019

Notes on graph
- Program was made available in April 2009.
- There was no tracking system in place from Jan 1, 2015 until July 15, 2017.
- Not all children doing HP in North America are registered with FHCi.
- Not all who enrolled with FHCi have completed the program.
- Total accounted for as of December 31 2019 = 1511.

Introduction

References*

*References in the following articles are numerically in continuation from this section

i.   Gaithersburg, MD. "Vaccines and Related Biological Products Advisory Committee." FDA Center for Biologics Evaluation and Research. 2010-05-07.

ii.   Hooper, Edward. "The River: A Journey to the Source of HIV and AIDS." Boston: Back Bay Books, 2000.

iii.   Scheibner, Viera, PhD. "Adverse Effects of Adjuvants in Vaccines." Nexus 12-2000 & 2-2001.

iv.   Generation Rescue, Inc. "Autism and Vaccines Around the World: Vaccine Schedules, Autism Rates, and Under 5 Mortality." Rescuepost.com. April 2009. Generation Rescue. http://www.rescuepost.com/files/gr-autism_and_vaccines_world_special_report1.pdf.

v.   Harris, Gardiner. "Deal in an Autism Case Fuels Debate." New York Times. March 2008.

vi.   Prevalence of Autism Spectrum Disorder Among Children Aged 8 Years — Autism and Developmental Disabilities Monitoring Network, 11 Sites, United States. 2016. https://.www.cdc.gov/mmwr/volumes/69/ss/ss6904a1.htm?s_cid=ss6904a1_w.

vii.   Hahnemann, Samuel. "The Cure and Prevention of Scarlet Fever." Lesser Writings. B Jain Publishers, New Dehli. Bracho, G, Varela, E.,Fernandez, R., et al. "Large-scale application of highly-diluted bacteria for Leptospirosis epidemic control." Homeopathy. 99 (2010): 156-166.

viii.   Bracho, G, Varela, E.,Fernandez, R., et al. "Large-scale application of highly-diluted bacteria for Leptospirosis epidemic control." Homeopathy. 99 (2010): 156-166.

ix.   Hahnemann, Samuel. "Organon of the Medical Art." Ed. Wenda Brewster O'Reilly. Palo Alto: Birdcage, 1996.

x.   Ibid.

xi.   Ibid.

xii.   Hahnemann, Samuel. "The Cure and Prevention of Scarlet Fever." Lesser Writings. B Jain Publishers, New Delhi.

xiii   Montagnier, Luc, et al. "Electromagnetic Signals are Produced by Aqueous Nanostructures Derived from Bacterial DNA Sequences." Interdisciplinary Sciences: Computational Life Sciences. 1 (2009): 81-90.

xiv.   Ibid.

xv.   San Diego Pathologists (2009). Certificate of analysis. https://freeandhealthychildren.org/certification-in-homeoprophylaxis/hpdocuments/remedy-sources/.

xvi.   Christine Stabell Benn. How vaccines train the immune system in ways no one expected. TEDxAarhus. https://www.youtube.com/watch?v=_d8PNlXHJ48.

xvii.   Birch, Kate, Glyphosate Free. KDP Publishing, USA, 2019.

Glossary of Terms

Antidote: When the action of the remedy is stopped short by some external means. In some individuals, certain substances have been known to interrupt the remedy action. Antidoting factors are also dependent upon how much time has passed since the person took the remedy before being exposed to an antidoting agent. Substances which have been known to antidote remedies are as follows: coffee, mint, strong smelling oils, tea tree oil, rosemary oil, camphor, eucalyptus. Remedies can also be antidoted if the person is exposed to electrical charges, such as electric blankets, dentist drilling, airplanes, radiation, or x-rays. Remedies can also be rendered ineffective prior to consumption if exposed to sunlight, high temperatures, radiation, strong smells, moisture, getting wet, touching or spilling the pellets on the floor.

Dose: An amount of remedy to be taken at one time (i.e., 2-5 pellets of a single remedy). Repeating the remedy means repeating the dose. Single dose means give 2-3 pellets once. Split dose means to repeat the 3 pellets once shortly after, anywhere from 5 minutes to 24 hours. Extended dose is to repeat in successive intervals over several hours. Triple dose refers to repeating the remedy 3 times in 24 hours.

Homeoprophylaxis (Homoeoprophylaxis)(HP): Use of a homeopathic remedy for the purpose of preventing disease. Remedies are not chosen according to symptom similarity of the person but rather as to their direct relation with the disease in question. Homeoprophylaxis (HP) can be achieved with a nosode (see below) of the disease or a single remedy that is known to have a particular affinity for that disease. (i.e., ***Belladonna*** for scarlet fever, ***Lathyrus sativus*** for polio, ***Ledum*** for tetanus, etc.)

Homeopathy: Derived from the terms 'Homeo' which means similar and 'Pathos' which means suffering/pathology. Refers to the practice of medicine where an agent that can cause a set of symptoms has the ability to cure that same set of symptoms.

Nosode: A homeopathic attenuation and dilution of pathological organs and/or tissues, causative agents, or disease products from infected individuals such as discharges, excretions, secretions, or pathological tissues.

Pilule/Pellet: Refers to the actual round white pellets given throughout the HP program.

Potency: Potency refers to the number of times a remedy has been diluted and succussed as per the definition of potentizing below. I.e. the remedies in this program are in a 200C and 10M potency. It means that they have been diluted and succussed 1 to 100 drops - 200 times or 10,000 times, respectively.

Potentizing: The process of repeated dilution and succussion in the making of a homeopathic remedy.

Remedy: Any substance that has been potentized according to the Homeopathic Pharmacopeia of the United States (HPUS). A homeopathic remedy is a medicament that can produce, in a healthy person, symptoms similar to the symptoms a sick person is experiencing. A remedy is only homeopathic if it is used according to homeopathic principles, regardless of potency.

Remedy Action: Refers to the drug action upon the body and the response of the body to the remedy. The greater the susceptibility the person has to the remedy, the greater its likelihood to cause a response. Therefore, the desired effect after taking a homeopathic remedy is the *Remedy Action* as the remedy is resonating with the body and stimulating it to respond. Remedies, which do not have any affinity to an individual, will not produce an action. In accordance with homeopathic principles, remedies are employed to enhance the healing mechanism of the body. There are no side-effects of the remedy other than the overall beneficial effects of mild immune response. After consumption of a remedy there may be an aggravation of existing conditions, but if a remedy has the ability to aggravate a condition it has an equal and opposite ability to ameliorate that same condition.

Titer: An antibody titer is a measurement of how much antibody an organism has produced in relation to an antigen (pathogen). The ELISA Western blot test is a common means of determining antibody titers. HP does not necessarily produce antibodies as we are stimulating the general immune system (the ability to produce a fever and discharge) rather than targeting specific antibody production.

                    Glossary of Terms

1. Establishing Homeoprophylaxis as a Public Healthcare Model

Key words: Homeoprophylaxis, Vaccination, Unvaccinated, Research, Leptospirosis, Nosodes, Public Health Programs.

By Kate Birch, RSHom(NA), CCH

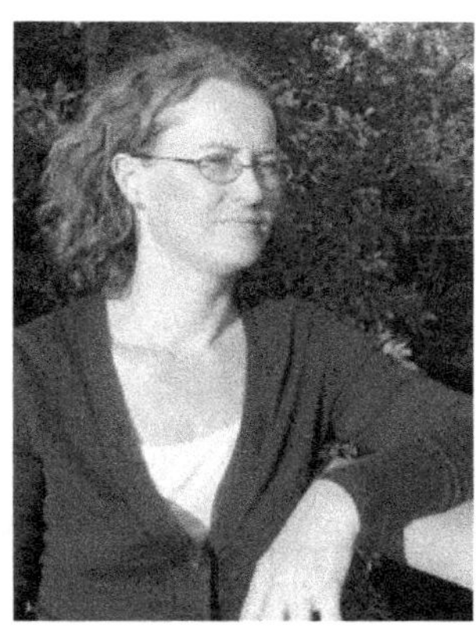

I never planned to be a researcher or an author, but in 2003 I became overwhelmed with the number of children in my practice who suffered from vaccine damage. I wanted to show the public that there were alternatives to vaccines and antibiotics. In 2007 I published, **Vaccine Free Prevention and Treatment of Infectious Contagious Disease with Homeopathy**.[xviii] In it I sought to condense the collective knowledge in homeopathy regarding infectious disease. The book's publication led me to be regarded as an international expert and teacher about homeopathy and contagious disease, such that In December of 2008 I was invited to speak at an international conference in Havana, Cuba. My paper was *The Role of Government in Infectious Disease Prevention*.[xix]

The international Convention on Homeoprophylaxis (HP) was held by the Carlos J. Finlay Institute (a Cuban World Health Organization-approved vaccine manufacturer). **NOSODES2008**[xx] was an "International meeting on homeoprophylaxis, homeopathic Immunization and nosodes for epidemics," which hosted representatives from twelve different countries speaking on a variety of programs, all reporting the efficacy of homeoprophylaxis and homeopathic treatment for infectious disease.

The central thesis of my paper was that it is the role of government to establish public health measures concerning infectious disease expression, and that the responsibility of government extends to understanding the beneficial role of certain diseases in human evolution, to establish programs that acknowledge the concept of collective susceptibilities, and to target safe and effective immunization programs towards those susceptibilities. Furthermore, these governmental public health measures should be motivated and directed by the notion of public good, i.e. a benevolence towards its citizens. Needless to say, such policies should also be grounded in the understanding of collective susceptibility, but also in an understanding that infectious disease incidence is directly related to not only sanitation but to socio-economic pressures as well. From that place of benevolence, it is the role of the government to address the socio-economic factors that contribute to infectious contagious disease expression.

Infectious disease occurs when there is an adaptive mechanism needed in that population. For example, the 1918 flu pandemic came immediately post World War I where the whole of humanity suffered a kind of shock or bereavement. The adaptive mechanism brought on by the influenza virus leads to humans caring for each other to heal some of that trauma. Common symptoms of that flu epidemic were a sudden onset and collapse and were correspondingly treated by *Gelsemium* which not only addresses flu conditions but also ailments from shock. If the infective process is denied through preventive intervention that does not address this susceptibility, we suppress that natural adaptation mechanism needed to heal the imbalance. The diagram below depicts this trajectory, or bell curve of evolution through a population. This comes from the understanding that all infectious diseases, but especially childhood infectious diseases, often serve to activate adaptive measures within the individual.[xxi] Additionally, traditional injected vaccinations, do not satisfy the healthy immunological development processes of individuals in the same way natural disease processes do. Furthermore, the introduction of a complex formulation of disease antigens, immunomodulators (adjuvants), antibiotics, and a host of other ingredients, generates a number of aberrant immunological responses and conditions.

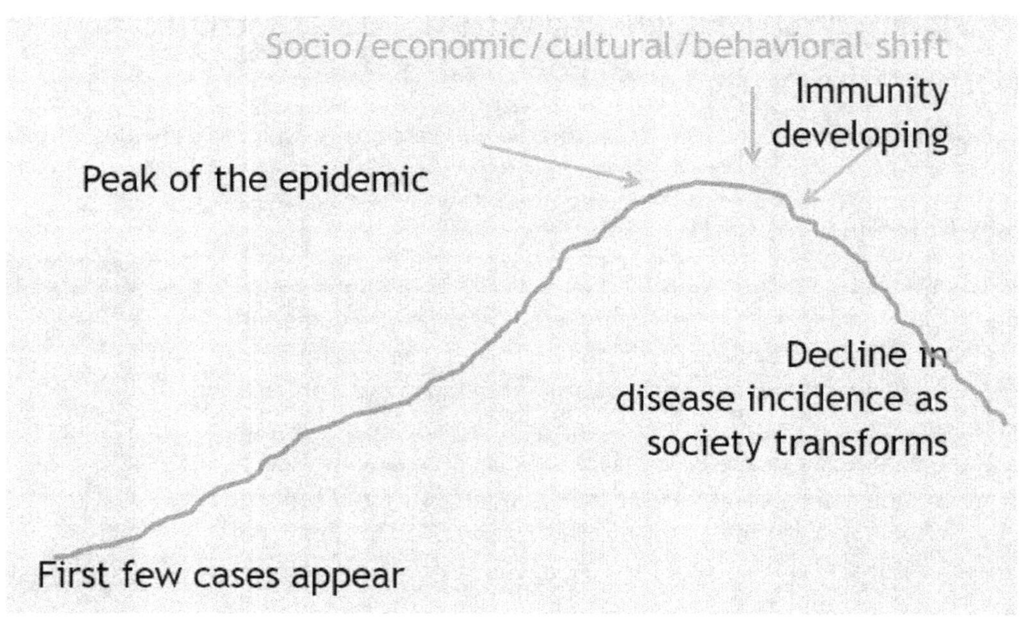

Figure 4. Bell curve of infectious disease over time in the general population

One of the more outstanding papers presented at the Cuba conference was by Isaac Golden, PhD, D.Hom., N.D., of Australia, who presented the results of the world's largest long-term study of homeoprophylaxis for childhood infectious contagious diseases.[xxii] Some 3000 individuals, over 15 years participated in his HP program. He found that the efficacy of HP was higher than that of vaccination. Furthermore, his results demonstrated that children who underwent the program were also statistically healthier than both those who were vaccinated -- and healthier also than those who received no treatment or prevention at all.[xxiii]

At that moment I realized that HP could be an alternative form of infectious disease prevention to vaccines. I decided that in order to establish homeoprophylaxis as a viable option in the United States I had to replicate Golden's research. I had little notion of the many steps needed to realize this.

As the Cuba conference progressed, and speaker after speaker presented papers on HP for infectious disease, it was obvious that tangible and successful methodologies already existed to apply homeoprophylaxis. Over the following ten years, this realization inspired me to develop and promote our research, education, and a mechanism of access to homeoprophylaxis.

Cuba's public medical system has long been extolled as one of the world's best. One ongoing issue that the Cuban Health Ministry had struggled with was the national and regional incidence rates of leptospirosis. Since 1981, the Health Ministry observed incidence rates rise and fall in response to rainfall, flooding and other natural disasters. The Finlay Institute had developed a vaccine for leptospirosis, but despite its use, disease incidence had remained flat. A more proactive effort needed to be made. In 2007 the Cuban Health Ministry opted for an HP trial with the assistance of the Finlay Institute, under the direction of Dr. Gustavo Bracho and Dr. Conception Campa Huergo, widely respected vaccine researchers and creators of the first ever meningococcal vaccine.[xxiv]

In 2007 and 2008, as Cuba was struck by a series of hurricanes, Noel, Dean, Gustav, and Ike respectively, the Direccion Nacional de Medicina Natural y Tradicional (Cuba), enacted studies of the homeopathic prophylaxis of leptospirosis.[xxv] The Health Ministry decided to inoculate three of the most vulnerable eastern provinces of Cuba with *noso*LEP, (a homeopathic preparation of four strains of leptospirosis). The remainder of Cuba was used as the research control population.

     Establishing Homeoprophylaxis as a Public Healthcare Model

When results were collected, it was shown that over the same time period, leptospirosis incidence in the HP regions had been reduced by 84%, while the rest of Cuba saw cases rose by 21% in the second year of the intervention.[xxvi]

In the following years the Finlay Institute continued its research on HP for leptospirosis. Since the initial large-scale interventions in 2007 and 2008, the incidence of leptospirosis has remained low in not only the three provinces given nosoLEP, but remarkably, *leptospirosis levels in the untreated population also retreated throughout the island.*[xxvii] This shift provides strong evidence that a shift in susceptibility to leptospirosis had taken place in the entire population, despite not everyone receiving the prophylaxis. Jeremy Sherr calls this a posi-demic.[xxviii] This idea concurs with the concept that collective susceptibilities are present in populations and that epidemic disease operates under this mechanism as do collective healings, or the idea that doing a proving in a group of people has the potential to effect collective consciousness. In this case inoculation in a large number of people with nosoLEP changed the entire population

Subsequent research has begun to clarify how HP impacts the immune system and antibodies. Research results comparing the effects of leptospirosis vaccine with HP have shown that while injection with vaxSPIRAL (the vaccine for leptospirosis) created antibodies in all mice recipients, with no mortality, oral introduction of nosoLEP (HP)--the same nosode used in prevention in humans--led to an 80% survival rate with no antibodies being produced. Based on these findings Dr Bracho's conclusion is that unlike the vaccine, nosoLEP activates cell-mediated immunity (that of the general immune system) rather than humoral immunity (antibody production).[xxix]

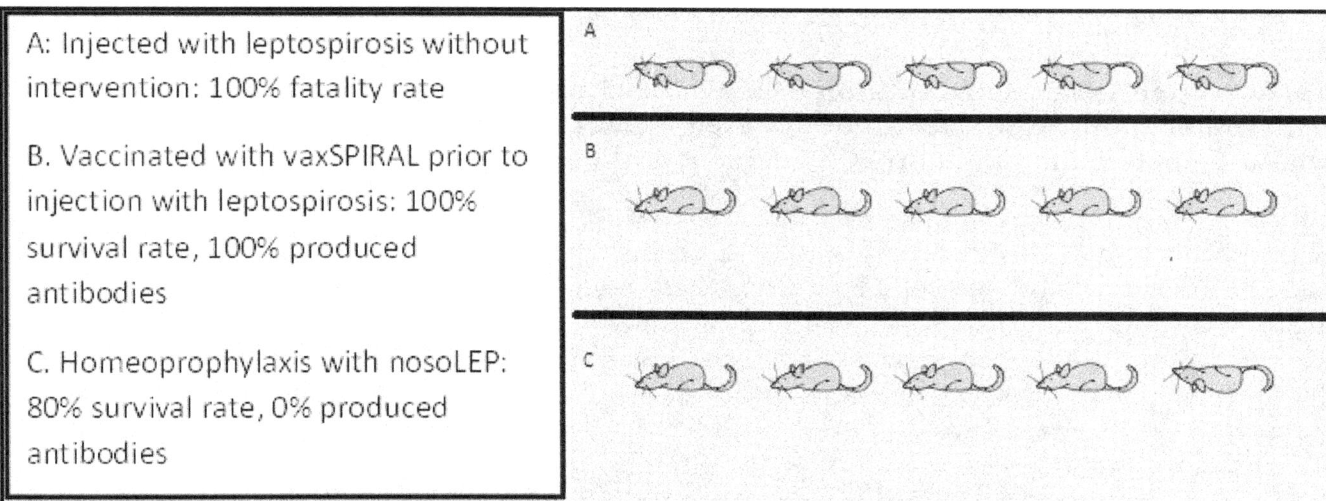

Figure 5. Research with antibody production in mice with nosoLEP

I was struck both by the level of coordination established by the Cuban government, and the generally humane and elevating sentiment I had seen its representatives express towards the health of its people. The attitude of the people implementing the study was that they were doing what they could to minimize infectious disease with homeoprophylaxis because it was *a gentle, non-toxic system of disease prevention.* The simple trust the people had in their government and their compliance with the intervention was a direct result of these attitudes on the part of the government. I took inspiration from these attitudes in developing my own next steps.

After investigating HP on my own, I found numerous studies around the world that had demonstrated the effectiveness of HP in a variety of diseases:[xxx] meningitis,[xxxi] polio,[xxxii] cholera,[xxxiii] dengue,[xxxiv] and diphtheria.[xxxv,xxxvi,xxxvii]

With increasing public concern over possible lack of safety of vaccination, and with copies of Isaac Golden's research paperwork and his blessing, I designed an HP study, trained other homeopaths in HP, and developed networks for HP access in North America.

In the United States, public health sentiments are vastly different than in Cuba. Since the inception of the National Childhood Vaccine Injury Act (NCVIC) of 1986,[xxxviii] and under the influence of the CDC, vaccine manufacturers, and other political powers, an ever-increasing vaccine schedule has emerged with seemingly little to restrain it. Concurrently autism rates have also increased since the 1980s: from 1-2 in 10,000, to 1 in 150 in 2000, to 1 in 69 in 2008, and to 1 in 59 in 2014.[xxxix,xl,xli] The CDC ceased reporting autism rates after 1014. Furthermore, in the last ten years numerous directives have sought to remove religious and medical vaccine exemptions through legislative mandate for vaccination state by state.[xlii,xliii] These mandates are promoted as government protecting the health interests of the populous, but if vaccines were as safe and effective as purported, people would participate without coercion and mandates. Over $4 billion has been paid out for vaccine injury and death,[xliv] while debates about whether HP is homeopathy or not continue to smolder in the homeopathic community.

With increased public concern regarding vaccines, and studies of their effects,[xlv] parents are actively seeking out alternative methods of disease prevention. Many are looking to HP as an alternative to the regular vaccine schedule.

To fulfill these needs, and in order to apply HP on a large scale, in 2011 Free and Healthy Children International (FHCi), a 501 (c) 3 charitable organization, was born.[xlvi] In 2019 and 2020 the 10 year-long study summarized below was published.

FHCi started with the inspiration of a model of application to follow, and an act of benevolence toward the health of children because of the absolute belief that HP would be better than the current vaccine paradigm.

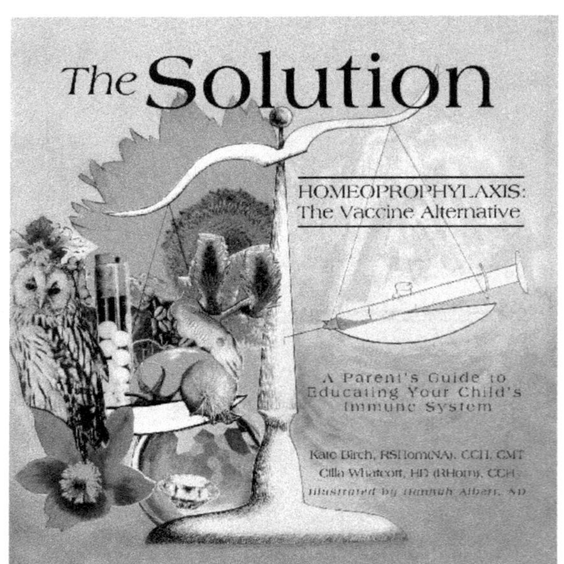

To promote understanding of the effectiveness and efficacy of HP, my former colleague, Cilla Whatcott, and I wrote the book, **The Solution Homeoprophylaxis: The Vaccine Alternative.** The aim of the book was to help parents understand how HP works in the developing immune system, but the book was also integral to educating homeopaths. We also attended courses from the National Institute of Health (NIH) on Research in Human Subjects as Principal Investigators.[xlvii] All of the NIH ethical parameters with regards to research were observed throughout registration and follow-up of our studies, and FHCi developed its own Adverse Event Reporting System and specific standards of ethical practice in HP.

In 2009 the initial parameters of the research had been developed and the first families seeking out HP were registered. In 2013 an application was made with attending documentation, overview, and waiver forms--to the Independent Review Board (IRB) of the American College of Homeopathy and the University of Phoenix Extension. This application was denied by the IRB due to assessment that the project was too large and inadequately funded. Despite this, the FHCi Board made an executive decision to continue with the research and program that we had implemented, as the urgency to produce more HP research in the face of increasing vaccine schedules and evidence of collateral damage was growing.

In 2018 a call for surveys and records was made. In the summer of 2019 two 5000+ - word abstracts were readied for publication. In 2020 and beyond, FHCi will promote these publications to the general public. We will also reflect on how best to present our work to legislative bodies with the goal of establishing homeoprophylaxis as a public health option. The current climate regarding the FDA and the revised draft guidance document which expressly identifies remedies with infectious agents gives us some pause in timing of our publication.[xlviii]

In conclusion I am grateful for the opportunity to have participated in making this HP research a reality. I thank all past and present FHCi board members, practitioners, and families who participated in the process from 2009 until now and look forward to greater acceptance of HP in the future because of this work.

Abridged summaries of the research:

1. Long-term homoeoprophylaxis study in children in North America. Part One: Factors contributing to the successful completion of sequential dosing of disease nosodes. [xlix]

2. Long-term homoeoprophylaxis study in children in North America. Part Two: Safety of HP, review of immunological responses, and effects on general health outcomes. [l]

By Kate Birch, RSHom(NA), CCH, Su Sandon, RPh, RSHom(NA), CCH, HMC, Sarah Damlo C.Hom, and Kim Lane, MD.

For the full abstracts please refer to the published articles.

The homoeopathic nosodes used over a period of 44 months included those made from whooping cough, mumps, measles, pneumonia, meningococcal disease, tetanus, and Haemophilus influenzae type B. Lathyrus sativus, a plant remedy with historical success in the prevention and treatment of polio, was used for polio.[li] Remedies were given in sequence according to the schedule outlined. Registration included health status of the child, age, and previous vaccine history if any. Fees for HP registration were paid for by the parents. Each child was equipped with a program booklet, HP kit, and directions. Parents were informed that there could be immune responses generated from the doses given and that these responses were intended to help develop the child's immune system.[lii] Response surveys were to be voluntarily submitted at various stages of the program. Limited resources and a passive tracking system significantly affected the response rate. Between 2009 and 2014, 56 HP supervisors collectively registered 682 children, between newborn and 10 years of age, of which 339 responded with surveys.

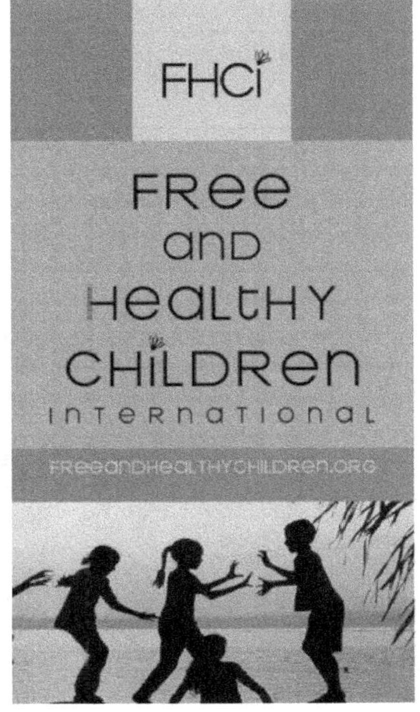

Part one was to determine if the social-economic profiles, past vaccination status, and health profiles of participants choosing HP had an effect on completion of a self-administered 44-month program.[liii] Part two was to determine the number and type of responses to HP remedies in *Unvaccinated* and *Previously Vaccinated* children and effects on general health outcomes. As 90% of the work that went into this research was voluntary and resources were spread over 15 states and 4 countries, the study of infectious disease incidence and contraction rates had too many confounding factors, and so were not meaningful, and have not been published at this time.

We also learned that HP activates an immune system response. These responses were mild and short lived. From this immune process the general health profiles for a variety of conditions improved, from registration to completion of the program.[liv]

Part One Summary

Table 1.1.a. references total number of participants, the gender of registrants, and number of *Unvaccinated* and *Previously Vaccinated* children at all levels of completion of the program. Of the 682 children registered, 126 *Completed*, and 62 *Completed in 50 months*. Upon registration 475 were *Unvaccinated* and 207 were *Previously Vaccinated*.

	Girls	Boys	Unspec	Totals	Unvaccinated	Previoulsly vaccinated
1. Total registered	330	341	11	682	475	207
Percentage of total	48	50	2	100	70	30
2. No contact	155	180	8	343	243	100
Percentage of total	45	52	2	100	71	29
Total respondants	175	161	3	339	226	113
Percentage of total repondents	52	47	1	100	67	33
3. Withdrew	15	19		34	21	13
Percentage of repondents	44	56		100	62	38
4. Started and Stopped	33	35	3	71	49	22
Percentage of repondents	46	49	4	100	69	31
5. 200C series	33	36		69	42	27
Percentage of repondents	48	52		100	61	39
6. 200C and 10M	29	10		39	23	16
Percentage of repondents	74	26		100	59	41
7. Completed	65	61		126	91	35
Percentage of repondents	52	48		100	72	28
8. Completed in 50 months	31	31		62	47	15
Percentage of completed	50	50		100	76	24

Table 1.1.a. Total number, gender, and previous vaccination status of registrants at all levels of completion

Part One Results: Of the 682 children initially registered, 50% had no contact due to a poor document tracking system. Of the 37% who *Completed*, 49% *Completed in 50 months*. 21% *Started and Stopped*, and 10% *Withdrew*. The degree of program completion was consistent with all ages. Children whose parents had undergraduate degrees, with incomes between $30,000-$50,000 (USD), and who never watched TV were more likely to complete the program. Time management issues and lack of understanding were identified as the two main obstacles to completion.

Part One Conclusions: We found that when middle class families of unvaccinated and partially vaccinated children understand what they are doing and are supported by competent practitioners, they are able to successfully complete this self-administered HP program. [iv]

 Establishing Homeoprophylaxis as a Public Healthcare Model

Part Two Summary

Table 2.1.a shows the total number of dosing series and actual doses administered compared to the number of responses per each dosing series given. In the program there are four dosing series for each remedy; 200c single dose, 200c triple dose, and 2 - 10M triple doses: for a total of ten individual doses per nosode. For one child to complete the program they would take 80 individual doses (ten doses of eght diseases). 35 of the 126 who responded as *Completed* did not provide a prophylaxis record. Their doses and responses are not included in these tallies. Accordingly, a total 140 dosing series and 350 individual doses are not included because the data was not verified.

	# of dosing series recorded	# of individual doses	# of responses recorded	% of responses for all series
Totals	3971	9333	597	15.03

Table 2.1.a. Total number of nosode/remedy responses as compared to dosing series recorded

Table 2.1.b. shows reported adverse events* compared to total number of dosing series per individual nosode/remedy. As per table 2.1.a. in a total of 9,333 individual doses given, there were no adverse events reported in both *Unvaccinated* and *Previously Vaccinated* cohorts.

* Adverse events as defined by the National Institute of Health guidelines for research on human subject is defined as a death, life-threatening adverse drug or device experience, inpatient hospitalization or prolongation of existing hospitalization, a persistent disability/incapacity, or a congenital anomaly/birth defect.[lvi]

	# of dosing series given	# of individual of doses	Adverse events reponrted
Pertussin	529	1255	0
Pneumococcinum	510	1204	0
Lathyrus sativus	497	1173	0
Haemophilus (Hib)	487	1145	0
Meningococcinum	490	1146	0
Tetanus Toxin	484	1130	0
Parotidinum	486	1140	0
Morbillinum	488	1140	0

Table 2.1.b. Adverse events repoted

Table 2.2 (facing page) compares frequency of conditions of the 126 children who *Completed in 50 months* in *Unvaccinated* and *Previously Vaccinated* cohorts to national incidence of each condition studied. The national data is collected from studies that took place approximately halfway through the time frame of the research 2009-2018 (half of the registrants entered the program in 2014; entrance closed December 31, 2014). National incidence for violence, fears, and mood swings are not referenced (facing page).

Summary of **Table 2.2**:

- 36.40% of *Previously Vaccinated* had ear infections upon registration. Incidence dropped to 18.20% by the completion of the program whereas national incidence was 57.8%. Ear infections in both cohorts were well below national averages.
- Seasonal allergies increased in *Unvaccinated*. Incidence of food allergies increased in *Unvaccinated* yet remained the same in *Previously Vaccinated*.
- Food allergies were higher than recorded national average in both cohorts.
- Food allergies increased in *Previously Vaccinated* during the program.
- Incidence asthma in both cohorts was below nation average and dropped in the *Unvaccinated*.
- Eczema was higher in both cohorts than national averages. Incidence of eczema rose from 15.40% to 19.10% in *Unvaccinated* and remained the same in *Previously Vaccinated*.

Final incidence in Learning disorders in *Completed* group.

3.a. Speech delay: 40% national, 6.4% *Unvaccinated*, and 4.5% *Previously Vaccinated*.

3.b. Disturbance in cognitive function: 15.4% national, 8.5% in *Unvaccinated* and 13.6% in *Previously Vaccinated*.

3.c. Disturbance in Social function: 20% national, 10.6% *Unvaccinated*, and 13.6 % *Previously Vaccinated*.

3.d. Neurological conditions: 10.7% national, 4.3% *Unvaccinated*, and 4.5% *Previously Vaccinated*.

	Unvaccinated registrants prior to HP	Unvaccinated HP recipients *Completed*	Previously Vaccinated registrants prior to HP	Previously Vaccinated HP recipients *Completed*	National incidence	Date	Title	Web link
1. General health								
a) Ear infections	16.20%	17.10%	36.40%	18.20%	57.8% 30%-80%	2016 2017	1. Ear Infection and Its Associated Risk Factors in First Nations and Rural School-Aged Canadian Children. 2. Otitis Media in Fully Vaccinated Preschool Children in the Pneumococcal Conjugate Vaccine Era.	https://www.ncbi.nlm.nih.gov/pmc/articles/PMC4764758/ https://www.ncbi.nlm.nih.gov/pmc/articles/PMC5751904/
b) Colds/sore throats/coughs	1 per year 31.2% 2 per year 22.5%	1 per year 15.0% 2 per year 37.0%	1 per year 50.0% 2 per year 22.7% 3 per year 9.1%	1 per year 27.3% 2 per year 27.3% 3 per year 36.4%	6/year average	2015	Viral aetiology of common colds of outpatient children at primary care level and the use of antibiotics	https://www.ncbi.nlm.nih.gov/pmc/articles/PMC3928210/
c) Seasonal allergies	10.5%	25.5%	18.20%	22.7%	11% 7.6%	2012 2017	1. Allergy: wikipedia 2. Summary Health Statistics: National Health Interview Survey	https://en.wikipedia.org/wiki/Allergy#Epidemiology https://ftp.cdc.gov/pub/Health_Statistics/NCHS/NHIS/SHS/2 017_SHS_Table_C-2.pdf
d) Food allergies: unspecified	14.7%	19.1%	35.4%	36.4%	10%. 6.5%	2014 2017	1. Food Allergy: Epidemiology and Natural History. 2. Summary Health Statistics: National Health Interview Survey	https://www.ncbi.nlm.nih.gov/pmc/articles/PMC4254585/ https://ftp.cdc.gov/pub/Health_Statistics/NCHS/NHIS/SHS/2 017_SHS_Table_C-2.pdf
e) Asthma	2.1%	0.0%	4.5%	9.1%	13% 10.8%	2017 2017	1. Summary Health Statistics: National Health Interview Survey 2. Summary Health Statistics: National Health Interview Survey	https://www.cdc.gov/nchs/fastats/asthma.htm https://ftp.cdc.gov/pub/Health_Statistics/NCHS/NHIS/SHS/2 017_SHS_Table_C-2.pdf
f) Eczema	15.40%	19.10%	18.20%	18.20%	12.97%%	2014	Associations of childhood eczema severity: A US population based study	https://www.ncbi.nlm.nih.gov/pmc/articles/PMC4118692/
2. Behavioral conditions			31.8					
a) Violence	8.4%	17%%	20.0%	13.6%			Data not found	
b) Mood swings	18.5%	31.9%	54.5%	50.0%			Data not found	
c) Fears	21.5%	36.2%	45.5%	40.9%			Data not found	
3. Learning disorders								
a) Speech delay	2.70%	6.40%	9.1%	4.5%	40%	2011	Communication skills in a population of primary school-aged children raised in an area of pronounced social disadvantage	https://onlinelibrary.wiley.com/doi/abs/10.1111/j.1460-6984. 2011.00036.x
b) Disturbance in cognitive function	2.3%	8.5%	9.1%	13.6%	15.04%	2008	Trends in the prevalence of developmental disabilities in US children, 1997-2008.	https://www.ncbi.nlm.nih.gov/pubmed/21606152
c) Disturbance in social function	4.6%	10.6%	9.1%	13.6%	20%	2006	Estimating the Prevalence of Early Childhood Serious Emotional/Behavioral Disorders: Challenges and Recommendations	https://www.ncbi.nlm.nih.gov/pmc/articles/PMC1525276/
d) Neurological conditions	2.50%	4.30%	0.0%	4.5%	10.70%	2013	Hospitalizations of children with neurological disorders in the United States	https://www.ncbi.nlm.nih.gov/pmc/articles/PMC3795828/

Table 2.2. Comparing frequency of incidence in general health outcomes of *Unvaccinated* and *Previously Vaccinated* to national incidence in those *Completed*.

Part Two Results: Of the 682 registered children, 475 were *Unvaccinated* and 207 were *Previously Vaccinated*. Of the total 339 respondents, 206 were *Unvaccinated* and 113 were *Previously Vaccinated* and had a total of 1,927 previous vaccine-disease doses. A total of 9,333 individual nosodes/remedy doses were given, which elicited 597 immune responses. Common responses included short-lived fevers, coughs, runny noses, restlessness or sleepiness, and perspiration with no adverse events reported. A full description of symptoms elicited are reviewed in the full abstract.

Incidence of general health conditions in *Unvaccinated* and Previously *Vaccinated* cohorts for all who completed the program improved in nearly all areas studied as compared to national incidence. Incidence remained below national averages in all neurological developmental parameters.

Part Two Conclusions: Results demonstrate that HP offers both unvaccinated and previously vaccinated children a low-risk immunization method that improves general health outcomes. Improved health outcomes in the previously vaccinated group suggests that HP may be of benefit after previous vaccination.

Economic disclosure of Free and Healthy Children International

(FHCi): 612-338-1668 FHCint@gmail.com, https://freeandhealthychildren.org/

1. Principle Investigator: Kate Birch, RSHom, CCH, 612-701-0629, katebhom@hotmail.com
2. Document Collection Person: Su Sandon, RPh, RSHom(NA), CCH, HMC, 612-889-2683 suhomeopathy@earthlink.net
3. Medical Advisor: Kim Lane, MD, 651-347-1952 wellnesslane@comcast.net

Data Entry:

4. Sarah Damlo, 952-212-3372, FHCigrants@gmail.com
5. Tana Harahan, 651-272-0932, FHCint@gmail.com
6. Katie Bromme, 612-327-3855, FHCiresearch@gmail.com
7. Max Sagert, 651-587-4047, FHCiresearch@gmail.com

Who	Total paid from 2009-2019 (USD)
Kate Birch	$4,815.00
Su Sandon	$6,865.77
Sarah Damlo	$3,885.00
Katie Bromme	$1,466.25
Max Sagert	$1,011.50
Tana Harahan	$670.00
Kim Lane	N/A
Total paid	$18,713.52

Figure 6. Economic disclosure for Part One and Two

Free and Healthy Children International (FHCi) is a 501(c)3 non-profit membership organization dedicated to research, education, and access to homoeoprophylaxis. It is registered for business in the state of MN, USA. From April 2009-December 2014, 682 children were registered in this research. From January 2015 to July 16, 2019 we did not have a tracking system in place. From July 17, 2017, to September 2019 an additional 1,044 children registered with FHCi.

We are independently funded by individual contributions and membership dues. All fees paid for organizing and tabulating the research were dispersed on either a quarterly stipend or hourly basis. There are no personal direct economic benefits derived from the results of this study. FHCi is not economically associated with any pharmacy that would benefit from the sale of the homoeopathic remedies utilized in this research. All research staff are homeopaths and live in the state of MN. We did this research because we are invested in the health of children. Thank you to everyone who helped this research come to fruition.

Homoeoprophylaxis is for free and healthy children!

References*

*Reference numeration continues from previous section.

xviii   Birch, Kate. "Vaccine Free Prevention and Treatment of Infectious Contagious Disease with Homeopathy." 2nd Edition. Germany: Narayana, 2010.

xix   NOSODES2008, "International Meeting on Homeoprophylaxis (HP), Homeopathic Immunization, and Nosodes for Epidemics." https://immunizationalternatives.com/wp-content/uploads/2015/05/Article_International_Meeting_On_Homeoprophlylaxis_Homeopathic_Immunization_and_Nosodes_Against_Epidemic_Diseases.pdf (Last viewed December 31, 2019).

xx   Ibid.

xxi   Adams, David. Rudolf Steiner on Traditional Childhood Illnesses and Vaccines. https://paam.wildapricot.org/resources/Pictures/07%20RS-Traditional%20Childhood%20Illnesses%20and%20Vaccines.pdf (Last viewed 4 October 2019).

xxii   Golden, Dr. Isaac. "Homeoprophylaxis – A Fifteen Year Clinical Study: A Statistical Review of the Efficacy and Safety of Long-Term Homeoprophylaxis." Isaac Golden Publications. Gisborne. Vic. 2004.

xxiii   Ibid.

xxiv   Carlos J Finlay Vaccine and Serum Institute. 2004. https://www.nti.org/learn/facilities/341/ (Last viewed 4 October 2019).

xxv   Bracho, G., Varela, E., Fernandez, R., et al. "Large-scale application of highly-diluted bacteria for Leptospirosis epidemic control." Homeopathy. 99 (2010): 156-166.

xxvi   Ibid.

xxvii   Bracho, Dr Gustavo, "Homeoprophylaxis: Evidences from Basic Research and Practical Applications." Homeopathic Research Institute (HRI), Barcelona. June 2013.

xxviii   Sherr, Jeremy. Homeopathy for Health in Africa. Homeopatia ahora. http://homeopatiaahora.blogspot.com/2009/04/homeopathy-for-health-in-africa.html (Last viewed 12/23 2019).

xxix   Bracho, Dr Gustavo, "Homeoprophylaxis: Evidences from Basic Research and Practical Applications." Homeopathic Research Institute (HRI), Barcelona. June 2013. (Last viewed 12/23 2019).

xxx   Clever, H (2015). Epidemiological studies in homeopathy. https://cleverhthemag.com/2015/12/01/epidemiological-studies-in-homeopathy/ (Last viewed 4 October 2019).

xxxi   Castro, D. and Nogueira, G. "Use of the nosode Meningococcinum as a preventative against meningitis." Journal of the American Institute of Homeopathy. 1975 Dec 68 (4), 211-219.

xxxii   Saine, Andre ND. "Homeopathic Prophylaxis in Epidemic Disease: History and Practice." Lecture notes: California, December 1988.

xxxiii   Thomas, William E, MD. "Asiatic Cholera Epidemic 1830 and Homeopathy." http://www.angelfire.com/mb2/quinine/cholera1830.html (Last Viewed Oct 4, 2019).

xxxiv   "Contribution of Homeopathy to the Control of an Outbreak of Dengue in Macaé," Rio de Janeiro Laila Aparecida de Souza Nunes Municipal Secretary of Health, Macaé, RJ, Brazil Int J High Dilution Res 2008; 7(25):186-192.

xxxv   Chavanon, P. La Dipterie, 4th edition. St. Denis, Niort: Imprimerie 1932.

xxxvi   Patterson, J and Boyd WE. "Potency Action: A Preliminary Study of the Alteration of the Schick Test by a Homeopathic Potency." British Homeopathic Journal 1941; 31: 301-309.

xxxvii   Eizayaga, F. "Tratamiento Homeopatico de las Enfermedades Agudas y Su Prevension." Homeopatia 1985; 51(342): 352-362.

xxxviii   The National Childhood Vaccine Injury Act (NCVIA) of 1986. https://en.wikipedia.org/wiki/National_Childhood_Vaccine_Injury_Act (Last viewed 4 October 2019).

xxxix   Autism Statistics. 2019. http://brighttots.com/Autism/Statistics.html (Last viewed 4 October 2019).

xl   Harris, Gardiner. "Deal in an Autism Case Fuels Debate." New York Times. March. 2008.

xli   Data & Statistics on Autism Spectrum Disorder. CDC. 2019. https://www.cdc.gov/ncbddd/autism/data.html (Last viewed 4 October 2019).

xlii   SB 2164. Title 6 Poliomyelitis and other diseases NY. June 13, 2019. https://www.health.ny.gov/prevention/immunization/docs/2164.pdf (Last viewed 4 October 2019).

xliii SB 277 CA. Public Health: Vaccinations. CA, 2015-2016. https://leginfo.legislature.ca.gov/faces/billNavClient.xhtml?bill_id=201520160SB277 (Last viewed 4 October 2019).

xliv Shilhavy, Brian. Uncensored: US Government Pays Out Over $4 Billion for Vaccine Injuries and Deaths. Health Impact News. Oct, 2019. https://healthimpactnews.com/2019/uncensored-us-government-pays-out-over-4-billion-for-vaccine-injuries-and-deaths/ (Last viewed 4 October 2019).

xlv Seneff, S. Glyphosate + aluminum + mercury + glutamate = autism. AutismOne Media. June 1, 2018. https://www.youtube.com/watch?v=OL9mr599hb0 (Last viewed 12/23 2019).

xlvi Free and Healthy Children International (FHCi). 612-338-1668. FHCint@gmail.com.

xlvii Human Subjects Research. https://grants.nih.gov/policy/humansubjects.html (Last viewed 4 October 2019).

xlviii Drug Products Labeled as Homeopathic: Guidance for FDA Staff and Industry. Revised Draft October 2019. https://www.fda.gov/regulatory-information/search-fda-guidance-documents/drug-products-labeled-homeopathic-guidance-fda-staff-and-industry (Last viewed 12/23 2019).

xlix Birch, K, Sandon, S, Damlo, S, Lane, K. Long-term homoeoprophylaxis study in children in North America. Part One: Factors contributing to the successful completion of sequential dosing of disease nosodes. Similia. Journal of the Australian Society of Homeopaths. Dec. 2019.

l Birch, K, Sandon, S, Damlo, S, Lane, K. Long-term homoeoprophylaxis study in children in North America. Part Two: Safety of HP, review of immunological responses, and effects on general health outcomes. Similia. Journal of the Australian Society of Homeopaths. June 2020.

li Sheffield, F (2014). Homeoprophylaxis: Human Records, Studies and Trials. https://www.homeopathycenter.org/news/homeoprophylaxis-human-records-studies-and-trials) (Last viewed 4 October 2019).

lii Adams, David. Rudolf Steiner on Traditional Childhood Illnesses and Vaccines. https://paam.wildapricot.org/resources/Pictures/07%20RS-Traditional%20Childhood%20Illnesses%20and%20Vaccines.pdf (Last viewed 4 October 2019).

liii Birch, K, Sandon, S, Damlo, S, Lane, K. Long-term homoeoprophylaxis study in children in North America. Part One: Factors contributing to the successful completion of sequential dosing of disease nosodes. Similia. Journal of the Australian Society of Homeopaths. Volume 31, Number 2, December. 2019.

liv Birch, K, Sandon, S, Damlo, S, Lane, K. Long-term homoeoprophylaxis study in children in North America. Part Two: Safety of HP, review of immunological responses, and effects on general health outcomes. Similia. Journal of the Australian Society of Homeopaths. Volume 32, Number 1, June. 2020.

lv Ibid.

lvi (1999). Guidance on reporting adverse events to institutional review boards for nih-supported multicenter clinical trials. National Institute of Health. US. https://grants.nih.gov/grants/guide/notice-files/not99-107.html (Last viewed 4 October 2019).

2. Long-term homoeoprophylaxis study in children in North America. Part One: Factors contributing to the successful completion of sequential dosing of disease nosodes*

Free and Healthy Children International HP Research Study-2009-2018.

Keywords: Children's Health, Developing Immune Systems, Homoeoprophylaxis (HP), Infectious Disease, Nosodes, Public Health Program, Unvaccinated, Vaccines.

By Kate Birch, RSHom(NA), CCH, Su Sandon, RPh, RSHom(NA), CCH, HMC, Sarah Damlo, C.Hom, Kim Lane, MD.

Abstract

Introduction: Currently the largest movements to curb and prevent infectious contagious disease in children are sanitary public health care measures and/or antibiotics and vaccines that carry inherent risks.[lvii,lviii,lix]

Individual adherence to public health programs is variable, based on education, economic standing, and confidence in those administering the program. Homoeoprophylaxis (HP) offers a low-risk infectious contagious disease prevention method to those parents looking for alternatives.[lx,lxi]

Method: The purpose of this study is to understand how best to implement and who are likely candidates for a self-administered 44-month long HP program. This is a long-term study using real-world participants who may have multiple diagnoses and needs. Part One reviews socio-economic factors that contributed to registration and successful study completion; it involved 682 healthy unvaccinated or partially vaccinated children between the ages of one month and 10 years old. Five percent of the children were over 10 years of age.

Results: This program appealed to two parent families with above average income and undergraduate or graduate education. Of the children registered, 69% were unvaccinated, while others opted for HP even after they had received a few vaccines or had completed several years of vaccines. 34% of the registrants were under the age of one year. The majority of children will or did attend public or private school, watch TV every day, and were omnivores.

Of the 682 children initially registered 50% we had *No Contact* due to a poor document tracking system. Of the 37% *Completed*, 49% *Completed in 50 months*. 21% *Started and Stopped*, and 10% *Withdrew*. Degree of completion of the program was consistent with all ages. Children whose parents had undergraduate degrees, with incomes between $30,000-$50,000 (USD), and never watched TV were more likely to complete the program. Time management issues and lack of understanding were the two main limitations to completion.

These results led to several program enhancements to promote greater success in program completion. Changes include not only the diseases covered and order of nosodes[lxii] in the program, but supplemental parent education and enhanced practitioner support. Collection of a more thorough initial inquiry into immune system readiness for HP from prenatal, birth, and previous vaccine histories will demonstrate if there is a need for homoeopathic treatment prior to commencing the program.

Conclusions: We have found that when middle class families of unvaccinated and partially vaccinated children understand what they are doing and are supported by competent practitioners they are able to successfully complete this self-administrated HP program.

* Nosodes are defined by the Food and Drug Administration's (FDA) Homeopathic Pharmacopoeia of the United States (HPUS) as homeopathic "attenuation of pathological organs and/or tissues, causative agents, or disease products from infected individuals, such as discharges, excretions, and secretions.

Introduction

Parent and HP Supervisor education was directed towards understanding the following principles: HP is not vaccination, nor a substitute for vaccination, but rather a form of immunisation that through the immune system responses generated, offers the possibility of gaining the benefits of natural acquisition of the disease by stimulating a mild, short lived, disease-specific response that activates the immune system towards immunity and enhances childhood development.[lxiii, lxiv]

The homoeopathic nosodes/remedies used in the HP Program include whooping cough, mumps, measles, polio, pneumonia, meningococcal disease, tetanus, and Haemophilus influenzae type B. Apart from polio, homoeopathic nosodes were used for each disease. For polio, Lathyrus sativus, a plant remedy with historical success in the prevention was used.[lxv] Parents were informed that there could be immune responses generated from the doses given and that these responses were intended to help develop the child's immune system.[lxvi]

Research Question

Part One: Are parents capable of completing a self-administered homoeoprophylaxis program within a set time frame for the purpose of preparing their child's immune system towards infectious disease processes?

Method

All children were registered between April 1, 2009 to December 31, 2014 under the supervision of a homoeopathic practitioner trained in HP (HP Supervisor). Once enrolled, they were to undertake a 44-month self-administered HP program, within 50 months, according to a previously set schedule for eight different diseases (see Prophylaxis Record following). At registration an Initial Health Profile and indication of the number of and type of vaccines previously given, if any, outlined the initial health of the child. Study design was based in part on the research by Dr. Isaac Golden.[lxvii]

Each family was equipped with:

1. An HP Program Booklet which included the Prophylaxis Record and HP Supervisor contact information.
2. A written comprehensive overview of the program.
3. Written instructions on how to complete the program.
4. A remedy dose/response journal.
5. Three questionnaires to be submitted at three different stages of the program.
6. An HP remedy kit. All nosodes/remedies in the kit were procured from the same registered homoeopathic pharmacy. Sources of nosodes serologically verified: all nosodes used were procured from active diseases in children collected between 2008 -2011 by San Diego Pathologists.[lxviii]

Parameters of Research

1. **Recruitment:** Passive registration through word of mouth, website searches,[lxix] and public lectures.
2. **Inclusion/Exclusion Criteria:** Inclusion and exclusion of participants was based on the following questionnaire: Inclusion was denoted by Yes's in first section, and No's in second section. Exclusion would include a negative to any one inclusion criteria. As there was interest in undertaking the program from overseas, we included them as well.

Inclusion Exclusion Criteria		
Yes	No	1. Questions
		As a parent do you have the desire to use an alternative infectious disease prevention method to vaccination?
		Do you reside in United States or Canada?
		Is your child under the age of eleven years old age for the proposed commencement date?
		Will you partake in the informed consent process?
		Will you be able to comply with follow up questionnaires?
		Do you have access to conventional or alternative medical care?
		Does your child display evidence of healthy immune function?
		2. Does or has your child need(ed) medication or treatment of any of the below conditions?
		Severe Allergies
		Severe Skin conditions
		Repeated illness (more than once a month)
		Developmental delay
		Behavioral difficulties
		Atypical Neurological Development

Figure 7. Inclusion/Exclusion criteria

3. **Consent:** An extensive Informed Consent process was completed for each participant. All Personal Health Information (PHI) was ethically collected and protected. All parents of subjects had the opportunity to review and sign consent forms prior to meeting with their HP Supervisors.

    These forms included the following points:
    1. Identification of sponsor: Free and Healthy Children International (FHCi)
    2. Identification of procedure
    3. Identification of risks and benefits
    4. Fees and compensation
    5. Withdrawal mechanism
    6. Confidentiality and release of Personal Health Information (PHI) notice
    7. Informed consent, parents sign
    8. Minors consent for children over the age of 6
    9. Minnesota (MN) HP Supervisor exemption waiver
    10. State or Provincial HP Supervisor waiver

4. **Data protection:** All registration and follow-up documents were submitted by mail to the Document Collection Person (DCP). Only the DCP, Principal Investigators (PI), and Data Analysis Team (DAT) had access to this information. Personal Health Information (PHI) will not be used or disclosed to a third party, except as required by law or permitted by authorised signature by the research subject: parent or guardian. All personal identifiers were held separate from data entries for research parameters. All hard copies of the data were kept secure and electronic versions password protected.

Publication of the data removes all personal identification of subjects except for the following:
1. Age
2. Geographical subdivisions such as state, province, or country
3. Health outcomes and nosode/remedy responses

5. **Control and Ethical Considerations:** In the study of infectious disease, it is unethical to deliberately expose study participants to infectious agents. Therefore, the control group used is infectious disease incidence in vaccinated and unvaccinated populations in the general public.

6. **Blinding:** There was no blinding method built into the study. All participants received the actual nosodes (or in the case of polio, Lathyrus sativus).

7. **Standardization of Treatment:** All subjects adhered to the HP program as delineated in Chart A. Prophylaxis Record, with dosing dates to be the first Sunday of the month. Adjustment of the program was possible if other needs of the child arose, such as, but not limited to the following:
    1. If there was an outbreak of a disease covered later in the program, that nosode/remedy could be administered earlier in the program.
    2. Supplemental nosodes could be added to the program in case of travel or disease outbreak. Responses to these remedies were not included in this data.
    3. If the child was sick at the time when a dose was to be taken, the dosing was postponed until one week after the sickness resolved. The following dose was to be given on time. If the parent forgot to give a dose, they were to give it as soon as they remembered and then continue with the program as scheduled on the first Sunday of the month. They were to wait at least two weeks from last HP dose before the next disease was introduced.
    4. If the parent gave one or two doses of the triple dose and forgot to give the second or third dose, they were instructed to give the entire triple doses series as soon as they remembered.

8. **Data collection:** All data generated was procured directly from the parents via passive submission of follow-up questionnaires. Call for submissions was announced through newsletters, email correspondence, and telephone contact. The questionnaires are as below.

1. Initial Socioeconomic Data to determine the following points:
a) Family type (married, single, other)
b) Yearly income
c) Highest education of parents
d) Medical insurance coverage
e) Education choices for the child
f) Dietary choices
g) TV use

2. Initial Health Profile parameters include:
1. Gender and age of child at registration
2. Previous vaccination
3. Previous infectious disease exposure and acquisition
4. Initial and ongoing health profiles
   a) Ear infections
   b) Colds/sore throats/coughs
   c) Seasonal allergies
   d) Food allergies
   e) Asthma
   f) Eczema
   g) Behavioral conditions
      i. Violence
      ii. Mood swings
      iii. Fears

Long-term homeoprophylaxis study in children in North America: Part one

h) Learning disorders
  i. Speech delay
  ii. Disturbance in cognitive function
  iii. Disturbance in social function
  iv. Neurological conditions

3. **Nosode/Remedy Dosing and Documentation:** All nosode/remedy responses were logged in the Remedy Journal provided.

4. **Cohorts:** Total registered and number of boys and girls in the following levels of completion of the program. The following cohorts were compared in tables reporting on:
   a. Age of entry into the program
   b. Prior vaccinations received
   c. Socio-economic standing of the family
   d. Reasons for incompletion of the program
   e. Accessibility to HP supervision and regional differences in completion of the program.

Cohorts identified in the following tables (numbers and definitions) (200C and 10M denote homoeopathic potency):
1. **Total registered:** Registered with an HP Supervisor by submitting informed consent form, initial health profile, and socio-economic data.
2. ***No contact:*** No follow-up paperwork was received, or the paperwork was sent and lost in the mail.
3. ***Withdrew:*** Submission of written notice of withdrawal from the program. Some may have given 1-3 doses before withdrawing.
4. ***Started and Stopped:*** A few doses in the first series were given and for a variety of reasons they stopped. They did not formally withdraw from the program but provided verbal or written notice of cessation of the program.
5. ***200C Series:*** Completion of the first 16 months of the program as documented by submission of the first questionnaire and/or Prophylaxis Record.
6. ***200C and first 10M series:*** Completion of the first 16 months and second 8 months of the program as documented by submission of the first and second questionnaires and/or Prophylaxis Record.
7. ***Completed:*** Completion of all stages of the program as documented by submission of the first, second, and third questionnaires and/or Prophylaxis Record.
8. ***Completed in 50 months:*** Completion of the 44-month program within 50 months by comparison of start dates and completion dates documented on questionnaires and/or Prophylaxis Record.

9. **Adverse Events:** An Adverse Event reporting procedure was developed to track any life-threatening or permanently disabling events. Remedy responses that mimic the normal symptoms of the disease are not considered adverse events but rather the desired immunological response. Responses that lasted more than 12-24 hours were reviewed and supported with additional dosing or if needed treated homoeopathically based on symptom presentation.

10. **Exit strategy:** Parents could opt out of the program at any time and if they wanted to pursue the use of vaccines they could at any time.

On the facing page is Chart A. Homoeoprophylaxis program (Prophylaxis Record)

Parents are to note the date of administration to be noted for each dose and check marks for responses which are to be logged in separate journal pages. One (1) month is either the age of the child at the onset of the program or first month of doses given.

Relationship between nosode and specific disease: ***Pertussin*** – Whooping Cough; ***Pneumococcinum*** – Pneumococcus; ***Lathyrus sativus*** – Polio; ***Haemophilus*** – Haemophilus influenzae Type B/Hib; ***Meningococcinum*** – Meningococcus, ***Tetanus toxin*** – Tetanus; ***Parotidinum*** – Mumps; ***Morbillinum*** – Measles.

Monthly Doses	Remedy	Potency	Label	Date	Initials	Check for response
1 month	Pertussin	200C	A1			
2 months	Pertussin	200C, 200C, 200C	A1			
3 months	Pneumococcinum	200C	B1			
4 months	Pneumococcinum	200C, 200C, 200C	B1			
5 months	Lathyrus sativus	200C	C1			
6 months	Lathyrus sativus	200C, 200C, 200C	C1			
7 months	Haemophilus (Hib)	200C	D1			
8 months	Haemophilus (Hib)	200C, 200C, 200C	D1			
9 months	Meningococcinum	200C	E1			
10 months	Meningococcinum	200C, 200C, 200C	E1			
11months	Tetanus Toxin	200C	F1			
12 months	Tetanus Toxin	200C, 200C, 200C	F1			
13 months	Parotidinum	200C	H1			
14 months	Parotidinum	200C, 200C, 200C	H1			
15 months	Morbillinum	200C	I1			
16 months	Morbillinum	200C, 200C, 200C	I1			
17 months	Rest or Supplemental Program					
Submit first questionnaire						

Monthly	Remedy	Potency	Label	Date	Initials	Response
18 months	Pertussin	10M, 10M, 10M	A3			
19 months	Pneumococcinum	10M, 10M, 10M	B3			
20 months	Lathyrus sativus	10M, 10M, 10M	C3			
21 months	Haemophilus (Hib)	10M, 10M, 10M	D3			
22 months	Meningococcinum	10M, 10M, 10M	E3			
23 months	Tetanus Toxin	10M, 10M, 10M	F3			
24 months	Parotidinum	10M, 10M, 10M	H3			
25 months	Morbillinum	10M, 10M, 10M	I3			
26 months	Rest or Supplemental Program					
Submit second questionnaire						

Monthly	Remedy	Potency	Label	Date	Initials	Response
28 months	Pertussin	10M,10M, 10M	A3			
30 months	Pneumococcinum	10M, 10M, 10M	B3			
32 months	Lathyrus sativus	10M, 10M, 10M	C3			
34 months	Haemophilus (Hib)	10M, 10M, 10M	D3			
36 months	Meningococcinum	10M, 10M, 10M	E3			
38 months	Tetanus Toxin	10M, 10M, 10M	F3			
40 months	Parotidinum	10M, 10M, 10M	H3			
42 months	Morbillinum	10M, 10M, 10M	I3			
44 months	Rest or Supplemental Program					
Submit third and final questionnaire						

Chart A. Homoeoprophylaxis program (Prophylaxis Record)

　Long-term homeoprophylaxis study in children in North America: Part one

Results

The tables below illustrate the number of children in various groupings and levels of completion in the program: review of gender, age, prior vaccination, socio-economic variables and access to HP Supervisors determine possible factors contributing to successful completion of the HP program.

Table 1.1.b. shows the total numbers and genders of children registered and at various completion levels of the program. Unspecified means that at registration the child was not yet born, or gender was never identified. The table indicates of the 34 that *Withdrew*, 15 were girls and 19 were boys representing 44% and 56% respectively of the total *Withdrew*.

	Girls	Boys	Unspec	Totals
1. Total registered	330	341	11	682
Percentage of total	48	50	2	100
2. No contact	155	180	8	343
Percentage of total	45	52	2	100
Total respondants	175	161	3	339
Percentage of total repondents	52	47	1	100
3. Withdrew	15	19		34
Percentage of repondents	44	56		100
4. Started and Stopped	33	35	3	71
Percentage of repondents	46	49	4	100
5. 200C series	33	36		69
Percentage of repondents	48	52		100
6. 200C and 10M	29	10		39
Percentage of repondents	74	26		100
7. Completed	65	61		126
Percentage of repondents	52	48		100
8. Completed in 50 months	31	31		62
Percentage of completed	50	50		100

Table 1.1.b. Total number of registrants and levels of completion: Comparing girls and boys

Table 1.2. identifies the number of children in different age groups compared to various levels of completion in the program. Percentages are relative to the number of respondents. For example, 24 % (82) of all the respondents were 0-6 months of age and 8% (27) of the total respondents *Completed* the program and were 0-6 months of age.

Age groups	1	2	3	4	5	6	7	8	Totals
Age in months	0 - < 6	6 - <12	12 - <24	24 - <36	36 - <60	60 - < 84	84 - < 120	120 +	
Age in Years	< .5	.5 < 1	1 < 2	2 < 3	3 < 5	5 < 7	7- <10	10 +	
1. Total registered	148	81	109	92	94	69	58	31	682
Percentage of total	21.70	11.88	15.98	13.49	13.78	10.12	8.50	4.55	100.0
2. No contact	66	47	52	51	43	41	29	14	343
Percentage of total	19.24	13.70	15.16	14.87	12.54	11.95	8.45	4.08	100.00
Total Respondents	82	34	57	41	51	28	29	17	339
Percentage of respondents	24.19	10.03	16.81	12.09	15.04	8.26	8.55	5.01	100.00
3. Withdrew	5	1	10	4	5	6	2	1	34
Percentage of respondents	1.47	0.29	2.95	1.18	1.47	1.77	0.59	0.29	10.03
4. Started and Stopped	18	6	13	8	14	7	5	0	71
Percentage of respondents	5.31	1.77	3.83	2.36	4.13	2.06	1.47	0.00	20.94
5. 200C series	20	7	10	9	9	7	3	4	69
Percentage of respondents	5.90	2.06	2.95	2.65	2.65	2.06	0.88	1.18	20.35
6. 200C and 10M	12	7	3	3	5	1	5	3	39
Percentage of respondents	3.5	2.1	0.9	0.9	1.5	0.3	1.5	0.9	11.50
7. Completed	27	13	21	17	18	7	14	9	126
Percentage of respondents	7.96	3.83	6.19	5.01	5.31	2.06	4.13	2.65	37.17
8. Completed in 50 months	11	11	6	10	9	3	6	6	62
Percentage of respondents	3.24	3.24	1.77	2.95	2.65	0.88	1.77	1.77	18.29

Table 1.2. Age groups of registrants

Table 1.3. shows the number of vaccine-disease doses of each disease recommended by the CDC. For example, in the first six months of life three doses of DTaP are recommended. DTaP has three diseases resulting in nine total vaccine-disease doses. When compared to Table 1.2, we can estimate the ages of the children in each group. Such as, of the 126 who *Completed* the program, as 13 children had between 24-41 doses of vaccine-disease doses, upon registration they were over 6 months old, had either stopped vaccinating after 24 months of age, or were not older than kindergarten age (maximum number of vaccine-disease doses for first 6 months is 23, at kindergarten is no more than 41). Two of the 126 had over 42 vaccine-disease doses which places them at 7th grade or older at time of registration. Ages of children at registration are tabulated in Table 1.2.

Each score represents one vaccine-disease dose	Birth to 6 months	12-24 months	At kinder-garten	7th grade	Total vaccine-disease doses
Hepatitis B	2	1	1		4
Diphtheria, Tetanus, Pertussis (DTaP)	9	3			12
Haemophislis influenza type b (Hib)	3	1			4
Pneumonia (PCV)	3	1			4
Rotavirus	2	1			3
Influenza	1	1	1	1	4
Polio (IPV)	3	1	1		5
Measles, Mumps, Rubella (MMR)		1	1		2
Chickenpox (Varicella)		1	1		2
Hepatitis A		2			2
Tetanus, Diphtheria, Pertussis (TDaP)				3	3
Meningococcal (MCV4)				1	1
Total doses per age group	23	13	5	5	46

Table 1.3. CDC early childhood immunisation schedule[lxx]

Table 1.4. shows us the absolute number of, and ranges of, the total number of previous vaccine-disease doses at each level of completion through the program. E.g., one DTaP vaccine contains three vaccine-disease doses. For example, we can see that 13 of the children who *Completed* the program had 24-41 vaccine-disease doses. Note: *Completed in 50 months* is a subset of *Completed*. When compared to Table 1.3., we can estimate the ages of the children in each range. Such as, of the 126 who *Completed* the program, 13 children had between 24-41 vaccine-disease doses, thus upon registration they at least were over six months old, had either stopped vaccinating after 24 months of age, or were not older than Kindergarten (max number of vaccine-disease doses for first six months is 23, at kindergarten is no more than 41). Two of the 126 had over 42 vaccine-disease doses which places them at 7th grade or older at time of registration. Ages of children at registration are tabulated in Table 1.2.

Ranges of number of vaccine disease doses	Total # of children	0	1 - 4	5 - 9	10 - 14	15 - 23	24 - 41	42 +	Total # vaccine-disease doses
1. Total number of vaccine-disease doses per child	682	469	62	29	17	31	56	18	3433
Percentage of 1.	100.0	68.8	9.1	4.3	2.5	4.5	8.2	2.6	
2. No contact	343	243	29	17	9	19	20	6	1506
Percentage of 2.	100.0	70.8	8.5	5.0	2.6	5.5	5.8	1.7	
Total respondants	339	226	33	12	8	12	36	12	1927
Percentage of respondents	100.0	66.7	9.7	3.5	2.4	3.5	10.6	3.5	
3. Withdrew	34	21	4	2	0	1	4	2	271
Percentage of 3.	100.0	61.8	11.8	5.9	0.0	2.9	11.8	5.9	
4. Started and Stopped	71	49	12	1	2	1	3	3	283
Percentage of 4.	100.0	69.0	16.9	1.4	2.8	1.4	4.2	4.2	
5. 200C series	69	42	5	4	2	2	13	1	447
Percentage of 5	100.0	60.9	7.2	5.8	2.9	2.9	18.8	1.4	
6. 200C and 10M	39	23	4	3	0	2	3	4	314
Percentage of 6.	100.0	59.0	10.3	7.7	0.0	5.1	7.7	10.3	
7. Completed	126	91	8	2	4	6	13	2	612
Percentage of 7.	100.0	72.2	6.3	1.6	3.2	4.8	10.3	1.6	
8. Completed in 50 months	60	47	2	1	3	2	4	1	255
Percentage of 8.	100.0	78.3	3.3	1.7	5.0	3.3	6.7	1.7	

Table 1.4. Total number of previous vaccine-disease doses per child at registration and at various stages of the program

Tables 1.5.a. -1.5.g. identify the socio-economic demographics of families who would choose HP. These variables are compared at each level of completion of the program. Income currency is USD.

a) Family type	Unspec.	Single parent	Married	Stepparent	GLBTQ	Other	Totals
1. Totals	34	26	596	4	2	20	682
Percentage	5	4	87	1	0	3	100.0
2. No Contact	17	11	299	3	0	13	343
Percentage of 2.	4.96	3.21	87.17	0.87	0.00	3.79	100.00
3. Withdrew	1	0	32	0	0	1	34
Percentage of 3.	3	0	94	0	0	3	100.0
4. Started and Stopped	2	7	58	0	1	3	71
Percentage of 4.	3	10	82	0	1	4	100.0
5. 200C series	8	0	60	0	0	1	69
Percentage of 5.	12	0	87	0	0	1	100.0
6. 200C, 10M	2	1	36	0	0	0	39
Percentage of 6.	5	3	92	0	0	0	100.0
7. Completed	4	7	111	1	1	2	126
Percentage of 7.	3.2	5.6	88.1	0.8	0.8	1.6	100.0
8. Completed in 50 Months	3	3	54	0	0	2	62
Percentage 8.	5	5	87	0	0	3	100.0

b) Yearly Income	Unspec	$0-$14,999	$5,000-$29,999	$30,000-$49,999	$50,000-$99,999	Over $100,000	Totals
1. Totals	57	12	71	112	256	174	682
Percentage	8	2	10	16	38	26	100.0
2. No Contact	27	10	38	59	111	98	343
Percentage of 2.	8	3	11	17	32	29	100.0
3. Withdrew	3	0	3	3	9	16	34
Percentage of 3.	9	0	9	9	26	47	100.0
4. Started and Stopped	7	0	9	15	26	14	71
Percentage of 4.	10	0	13	21	37	20	100.0
5. 200C series	8	0	5	7	37	12	69
Percentage of 5.	12	0	7	10	54	17	100.0
6. 200C, 10M	4	1	3	3	20	8	39
Percentage of 6.	10	3	8	8	51	21	100.0
7. Completed	8	1	13	25	53	26	126
Percentage of 7.	6	1	10	20	42	21	100.0
8. Completed in 50 Months	5	0	7	15	19	16	62
Percentage 8.	8	0	11	24	31	26	100.0

c) Highest education of parents	Unspec	High School	Undergrad	Grad	Tech School	Specialty	Totals
1. Totals	48	45	228	273	45	43	682
Percentage	7	7	33	40	7	6	100.0
2. No Contact	19	25	89	173	19	18	343
Percentage of 2.	6	7	26	50	6	5	100.0
3. Withdrew	5	4	17	4	1	3	34
Percentage of 3.	15	12	50	12	3	9	100.0
4. Started and Stopped	5	6	27	25	2	6	71
Percentage of 4.	7	8	38	35	3	8	100.0
5. 200C series	10	1	35	18	3	2	69
Percentage of 5.	14	1	51	26	4	3	100.0
6. 200C, 10M	4	2	12	10	7	4	39
Percentage of 6.	10	5	31	26	18	10	100.0
7. Completed	5	7	48	43	13	10	126
Percentage of 7.	4	6	38	34	10	8	100.0
8. Completed in 50 Months	3	3	26	21	3	6	62
Percentage 8.	5	5	42	34	5	10	100.0

d) Medical insurance coverage	Unspec	Don't have	Public assist	Private pay	Employee	Totals
1. Totals	56	61	81	153	331	682
Percentage	8	9	12	22	49	100.0
2. No Contact	30	34	44	87	148	343
Percentage of 2.	9	10	13	25	43	100.0
3. Withdrew	1	2	5	7	19	34
Percentage of 3.	3	6	15	21	56	100.0
4. Started and Stopped	7	5	9	15	35	71
Percentage of 4.	10	7	13	21	49	100.0
5. 200C series	10	8	0	12	39	69
Percentage of 5.	14	12	0	17	57	100.0
6. 200C and 10M	3	4	4	12	16	39
Percentage of 6.	8	10	10	31	41	100.0
7. Completed	5	8	19	20	74	126
Percentage of 7.	4	6	15	16	59	100.0
8. Completed in 50 Months	4	3	11	12	32	62
Percentage 8.	6	5	18	19	52	100.0

Long-term homeoprophylaxis study in children in North America: Part one

e) Education choice for the child	Unspec	Day care 1-12 months	Day care 1-3 years	Home School	Private School	Public School	Totals
1. Totals	83	31	73	164	192	139	682
Percentage	12	5	11	24	28	20	100.0
2. No Contact	38	14	33	99	92	67	343
Percentage of 2.	11	4	10	29	27	20	100.0
3. Withdrew	2	1	4	6	12	9	34
Percentage of 3.	6	3	12	18	35	26	100.0
4. Started and Stopped	10	3	8	15	21	14	71
Percentage of 4.	14	4	11	21	30	20	100.0
5. 200C series	13	6	6	13	26	5	69
Percentage of 5.	19	9	9	19	38	7	100.0
6. 200C and 10M	8	2	5	3	11	10	39
Percentage of 6.	21	5	13	8	28	26	100.0
7. Completed	12	5	17	28	30	34	126
Percentage of 7.	10	4	13	22	24	27	100.0
8. Completed in 50 Months	6	3	7	13	17	16	62
Percentage 8.	10	5	11	21	27	26	100.0

f) Dietary choice	Unspec	Vegan	Veg/ Eggs/ Dairy	Fish/ Chicken	Omnivore	Totals
1. Totals	70	12	32	84	484	682
Percentage	10	2	5	12	71	100.0
2. No Contact	34	0	12	25	272	343
Percentage of 2.	10	0	3	7	79	100.0
3. Withdrew	2	2	0	1	29	34
Percentage of 3.	6	6	0	3	85	100.0
4. Started and Stopped	12	1	1	1	56	71
Percentage of 4.	17	1	1	1	79	100.0
5. 200C series	9	3	3	10	44	69
Percentage of 5.	13	4	4	14	64	100.0
6. 200C and 10M	3	3	2	6	25	39
Percentage of 6.	8	8	5	15	64	100.0
7. Completed	10	3	14	41	58	126
Percentage of 7.	8	2	11	33	46	100.0
8. Completed in 50 Months	5	2	5	19	31	62
Percentage 8.	8	3	8	31	50	100.0

g) TV use	Unspec	Never	1-2 times a week	Every day	More than 3 hours/ day	Totals
1. Totals	51	159	192	273	7	682
Percentage	7	23	28	40	1	100.0
2. No Contact	24	75	100	144	0	343
Percentage of 2.	7	22	29	42	0	100.0
3. Withdrew	2	6	6	19	1	34
Percentage of 3.	6	18	18	56	3	100.0
4. Started and Stopped	8	15	19	29	0	71
Percentage of 4.	11	21	27	41	0	100.0
5. 200C series	7	15	23	22	2	69
Percentage of 5.	10	22	33	32	3	100.0
6. 200C and 10M	3	10	11	14	1	39
Percentage of 6.	8	26	28	36	3	100.0
7. Completed	7	38	33	45	3	126
Percentage of 7.	6	30	26	36	2	100.0
8. Completed in 50 Months	5	16	21	17	3	62
Percentage 8.	8	26	34	27	5	100.0

Tables 1.5.a.-1.5.g.: Socio-economic data of registrants in values and percentages

Table 1.6. Identifies limitations families had in completing the program. Data is from passive submission and confirmed by an additional survey and verbal confirmation. *Withdrawal* was notified in writing after 1-3 doses were administered. *Started and Stopped* included those who did several doses of various remedies but did not continue.

Any and all reasons per child/family included	
Total number who Withdrew (34) or Started and Stopped (71)	110
1. Time management issues unable complete the program	27
2. Did not identify the reason	20
3. Lost program	13
4. There were too many responses to HP doses	11
5. Never started	10
6. Did not have enough societal support. Feelings of isolation	9
7. Did not understand the program	6
8. Decided to vaccinate	5
9. Did not have the supervision needed to complete the program	4
10. Saving kit to see if there is an outbreak	4
11. Occupied by homeopathic constitutional care for ongoing health issues	4
12. Too many colds so couldn't do the doses	3
13. There were no titers produced when I tested so I stopped	3
14. No longer interested in doing the program	2
15. Developed eczema and allergies	1
16. Developed autism	1

Table 1.6. Reasons for Withdrew or Starting and Stopping

Table 1.7. identify the number and location (State, Province or Country) of HP Supervisors and children upon registration and at document tracking time. When cross-referenced they compare regional location completion of the program relative to number of active HP Supervisors.

1. Number of HP Supervisors per state or province at registration				1-3	4-7	18	Total
Total	0			19	19	18	56
Percentage	0.00%			33.93%	33.93%	32.14%	
Where				CO (1), FL (2), ID (2), IL (1), MA (1), ME (1), MI (2), NC (1), PA (1), TN (1), WA (2), WI (2), Japan (1), Portugal (1)	BC (7), CA (8), TX (4)	MN (18)	

1. Number of children per state or province at registration	0	1-4	5-14	15-29	30-73	301	
Total	0	57	106	59	159	301	682
Percentage	0.00%	8.36%	16%	8.65%	23.31%	44.13%	
Where		ALB (2), CT (2), DE (1), GA (4), HI (2), IA (4), IN (2), KS (2), MA (4), ME (4), MO (2), MS (1) NC (2), ND (3), NJ (2), NM (2), OR (1), QUE (2), SD (1), TN (1), UT (3), India (1) Japan (1), Mexico (2), Netherlands (4), United Kingdom (2)	AL (6), CO (7), ID (12), IL (13), LA (5), MI (9), NY (5), ONT (6), VA (5), WA (9), WI (14), WY (7), Portugal (8)	AZ (14), FL (29), PA (16)	BC (73), CA (56), TX (30)	MN (301)	

Table 1.7. Comparison of regional distribution of HP Supervisors and children at registration and upon completion of document tracking

Discussion

In 2009 this HP program was introduced to the public in the United States. At that time, parents of children of all ages and previous vaccination histories wanted to utilise it. Education of HP Supervisors in the management of HP was necessary to establish a mechanism of access to the program. At that time access to HP was only through registration in this research. The research was set up to rely upon passive submission of the data. In 2014 the main office for the receipt of data was moved. After one year the postal system ceased to forward the mail. Throughout 2018 we actively pursued the collection of questionnaires. A number of those early registrants contacted said that they submitted the only copy of their questionnaires in the mail, however, we did not receive them. Many had said they would send data, but they never did. Despite verbal communication with many of those categorised as *No Contact*, and even with verbal confirmation of progress and completion, without submitted paperwork we were not able to tabulate their results. Due to this poor tracking system 50% of registrant's did not submit any data. The numbers confirmed in these tables are from the received submissions. We expect that of those we did not receive data from, they share similar results to those that we did. The principal investigator registered 185 children, not only in the state of MN but around the country and internationally. Oversight of registered families and the other HP Supervisors in their management of the program reflect the results discussed below.

Gender of registrants: The program appealed equally to parents of both genders. Sex of the child does not appear to play a role in whether the parents were more likely to complete the program. There were a greater number of boys in the groups we *No Contact* or *Withdrew*. However, due to the small sample size we cannot draw any conclusions about compliance to the program with regards to gender.

Age of registrant: Those who started the program when the child was an infant or under the age of 12 months (Table 1.2, groups 1 and 2, 8% and 3.8% of total respondents, respectively) were more likely *Completed* and more likely *Completed in 50-months* (under 6 months - 3.2% and under one year - 3.2%). Group 3, children aged 12-24 months, were the next highest group in *Completed*. This trend was the same at all levels of progress in the program. In group 4 (ages 3-5) there are higher percentages of children who *Started and Stopped* or *Withdrew*.

Previous vaccination: Table 1.3. reviews the number of prior vaccine-disease doses. 69% of registrants had not received any vaccines indicating that HP was their preferred choice for disease prevention. As registrants were from all age groups this indicates that once awareness of HP was available parents wanted to participate in a public health care/disease prevention program regardless of the age of their child. For those who were introduced to HP with newborns or infants HP was their first choice, and others converted to HP from vaccination once they discovered this option. Of the registrants 31% had received prior vaccination: 9% of the total had 1-4 vaccine-disease doses, 8% had between 24-41 vaccine-disease doses, and 3% had more than 42.

One important variable was if the number of previous vaccines influenced motivation for completion of the program; 72.2% of the unvaccinated children *Completed* regardless of age. The next highest percentage of *Completed* was in children who had between 24-41 vaccine-disease doses. Causes identified for *Withdrew* or *Stopped and Started* were time management issues and irregular or prolonged immune system responses due to previous susceptibilities and the age of child. There were no adverse events reported. Additionally, successful completion of the program was dependent on support from HP Supervisors.

Conversion to HP: Conversations with registrants revealed that people turn away from vaccination for several reasons:

1. Adverse effects of vaccination.
2. They do not believe they work.
3. They do not like them.
4. They found HP as a safer more economical option.
5. They had started to vaccinate but then changed their minds either due to how their child responded to the vaccines or because of being introduced to HP.

Many families who *Completed* the HP Program had also completed the recommended vaccine schedule. Reasons for turning to HP include:

1. Wanting to introduce a more "natural" immunisation.
2. Doing HP might fix some of the effects on the child's health from the vaccines.
3. They did not have faith that vaccination actually did what is was purported to do.

Parents of unvaccinated children were more committed to the process of HP; 72.2% of those who *Completed* had no prior vaccines and 77.4% of those who *Completed in 50 months* had no prior vaccines. Additionally, as 10.3% of the total *Completed* had received 24-41 vaccine-disease doses, this indicates that despite previous vaccination their commitment to HP was equally high. We can also see that 18.8% of those who had only made it through the *200C Series* had between 24-41 vaccine-disease doses. One of the explanations for the delay in the program was the number of sicknesses the child experienced limited progression through the program, or there were too many responses generated. signifying that previous vaccine-disease doses increases susceptibility to acute disease or HP remedy responses.

Socio-economic influences: These tables show that at registration most parents were in the following categories:

a) Married.
b) The average annual income was between $50,000 and $99,000 (USD).
c) The highest level of education was university graduate.
d) They had employee paid health insurance (registration in the HP program was paid cash out of pocket).
e) They chose private school.
f) They were omnivores.
g) They watched TV every day.

Those *Completed* fit this profile:

a) Married.
b) Income $30,000-$50,000 (USD).
c) College undergraduate education.
d) Employee paid medical insurance.
e) Children went to public school.
f) They were omnivores.
g) Watched TV 1-2 times a week.

Household income of all levels of completion were from those who earned between $50,000-$99,999 (USD), except for 47% of the *Withdrew* who earned over $100,000 (USD). Considering that 42% of the children *Completed in 50 months* were from parents with undergraduate education may be reflective of the age group of the families with younger children were still in the process of their own education. TV usage is high in the *200 Series* and *200 and first 10M Series* and may be the lifestyle factor that limits time management and the successful completion of the program. 17% of day care usage in *Completed* demonstrates the number of children in that age group of registrants and the family's commitment to HP during these years of the child's development. Parents with younger children and the economic benefit of a middle-class lifestyle are more likely to complete the program.

Obstacles to completion: Time-management issues and confusion about responses to the nosodes were the biggest obstacles to completion of the program. Parents either did not communicate with their HP Supervisor or did not fully understand what the remedies were doing and were hesitant to give the next dose and were more likely to discontinue the program.

Program supervision: Table 1.7. informs us that those more likely to *Complete* lived in states/provinces where more HP Supervisors were offering HP and maintained membership with FHCi for the duration of the research. MN, BC (Canada), CA, and TX had the highest number of HP Supervisors and the highest number of registrants. This table verifies that response submission rates and completion of the program was more successful from families whose HP Supervisors were still with FHCi at the conclusion of the program. During these ten years not all the same HP Supervisors remained with FHCi; four that we know of passed away, three retired, and others changed the focus of their practice or realised they did not fully understand the process of HP to continue. Regional differences of registrants had to do with public awareness, acceptance of HP, and the ability to talk about it with their family and doctors. Since this program was established in Minnesota in 2009 public awareness has increased with regards to HP. Now some MN based medical doctors are happy to hear when families are doing HP if they are hesitant about vaccines. The net effect is a deeper commitment to the program. Conversely, the isolated registrants in those states or provinces where there was only one HP Supervisor undertook the program with little or no community support. Often parents of the same family were not in agreement and if there was a divorce, court orders more often sided with the parent who wanted to vaccinate. Subsequently, they dropped out of the program.

Next steps: In order to increase compliance and completion of the program an extensive review of those who discontinued was done. We cannot control individual participants, time management issues, nor family dynamics and the navigation through cultural beliefs and acceptance of HP. However, we can build community and influence public education and the expertise of our HP Supervisors. To build community we established a monthly-dosing-reminder newsletter and provided more ongoing information on what remedy responses mean. When we looked at the number of, intensity, and duration of remedy responses in the *Withdrew* and *Started and Stopped* cohorts, we opted to take more initial health information such as pregnancy issues, natural versus medical birth, and history of antibiotics and/or vaccines in both mother and child at registration to understand potential susceptibilities. With this information the goal is to provide more homoeopathic support prior to HP to prepare these children's immune system for homoeoprophylaxis.

Conclusions

Families want to participate in public health care programs. They want to invest in a low-risk disease prevention program that strengthens their children's immune systems. Growing distrust and increased risks of vaccinations are driving parents to look for alternatives. Completion of this program is possible for the typical middle-class family with average income and lifestyle choices. The largest obstacle to completing the program was the amount of time spent watching TV, perhaps contributing to time management issues. We have determined that when an HP family is well supported, they live in a community that is accepting of HP, and they can comprehend the process of immune system education with HP then they are more able to complete a self-administered HP program.

Economic disclosure

Sponsored by Free and Healthy Children International (FHCi). 612-338-1668 FHCint@gmail.com, https://freeandhealthychildren.org/.

1. Primary Investigator: Kate Birch, RSHom, CCH, 612-701-0629, katebhom@hotmail.com
2. Document Collection Person: Su Sandon, RPh, RSHom(NA), CCH, HMC, 612-889-2683 suhomeopathy@earthlink.net
3. Medical Advisor: Kim Lane, MD 651-347-1952, wellnesslane@comcast.net

Data Entry:

4. Sarah Damlo 952-212-3372, FHCigrants@gmail.com.
5. Tana Harahan, 651-272-0932, FHCint@gmail.com.
6. Katie Bromme, 612-327-3855, FHCiresearch@gmail.com.
7. Max Sagert, 651-587-4047, FHCiresearch@gmail.com.

Who	Total paid from 2009-2019 (USD)
Kate Birch	$3,290.00
Su Sandon	$6,865.77
Sarah Damlo	$3,685.00
Katie Bromme	$1,466.25
Max Sagert	$1,011.50
Tana Harahan	$670.00
Kim Lane	N/A
Total paid	$16,988.52

Free and Healthy Children International (FHCi) is a 501(c)3 non-profit membership organisation dedicated to research, education, and access to homoeoprophylaxis. It is registered for business in the state of MN, USA. From April 2009-Dec 2014 682 children were registered in research. From January 2015 to July 16, 2019 we did not have a tracking system in place. Since July 17, 2017, 1044 additional children have registered with FHCi. We are independently funded by individual contributions and membership dues. All fees paid for organising and tabulating the research were paid on either a quarterly stipend or hourly basis. There are no personal direct economic benefits derived from the results of this study. FHCi is not economically associated with any pharmacy that would benefit from the sale of the homoeopathic remedies utilised in this research. All research staff are homoeopaths and live in the state of MN. We did this research because we are invested in the health of children. Homoeoprophylaxis is for free and healthy children!

References*

*Reference numeration continues from previous section.

xli. World Health Organization (2018). Antimicrobial resistance. https://www.who.int/en/news-room/fact-sheets/detail/antimicrobial-resistance (Last viewed 26 September 2019).

xlii. Good, P (2018). Evidence the U.S. autism epidemic initiated by acetaminophen (Tylenol) is aggravated by oral antibiotic amoxicillin/clavulanate (Augmentin) and now exponentially by herbicide glyphosate (Roundup). Clinical Nutrition ESPEN. 2018 Feb;23:171-183. https://www.ncbi.nlm.nih.gov/pubmed/29460795 (Last viewed 26 September 2019).

xliii. Taylor, G (2018). 157 Research papers supporting vaccine/autism causation http://mainevaxchoice.org/wp-content/uploads/2018/10/VaccineAutismStudies.pdf (Last viewed 26 September 2019).

xliv. Golden, I (2004). The potential value of homoeoprophylaxis in the long-term prevention of infectious diseases, and the maintenance of general health in recipients. Graduate School of Integrative Medicine Swinburne University of Technology. https://immunizationalternatives.com/wp-content/uploads/2015/04/HP_Isaac_Golden_thesis_homeoprophylaxis1.pdf (Last viewed 26 September 2019).

xlv. Carmen (2012). Natural vaccine alternatives for you and your kids. Off the Grid News. https://www.offthegridnews.com/alternative-health/natural-vaccination-alternatives-for-you-and-your-kids/ (Last viewed 26 September 2019).

xlvi. Adams, D (2018). Rudolf Steiner on traditional childhood illnesses and vaccines. Our Spirit Reflections. https://neoanthroposophy.com/2018/03/01/rudolf-steiner-on-traditional-childhood-illnesses-and-vaccines/ (Last viewed 26 September 2019).

xlvii. Shefeild F (2019). Tutorial 6 – Provings. Can provings damage heath? Homeopathy Plus. https://homeopathyplus.com/tutorial-6-provings/.

xlviii. Clever, H (2015). Epidemiological studies in homeopathy. https://cleverhthemag.com/2015/12/01/epidemiological-studies-in-homeopathy/.

xlix. Adams, D (2018). Rudolf Steiner on traditional childhood illnesses and vaccines. Our Spirit Reflections. https://neoanthroposophy.com/2018/03/01/rudolf-steiner-on-traditional-childhood-illnesses-and-vaccines/.

lxvii Golden, I (2004). The potential value of homoeoprophylaxis in the long-term prevention of infectious diseases, and the maintenance of general health in recipients. Graduate School of Integrative Medicine Swinburne University of Technology. https://immunizationalternatives.com/wp-content/uploads/2015/04/HP_Isaac_Golden_thesis_homeoprophylaxis1.pdf.

lxviii San Diego Pathologists (2009). Certificate of analysis. https://freeandhealthychildren.org/certification-in-homeoprophylaxis/hpdocuments/remedy-sources/.

lxix Free and Healthy Children International. (Est 2011). https://freeandhealthychildren.org/.

lxx CDC Immunization Schedule (2014). https://www.cdc.gov/vaccines/schedules/index.html.

3. Long-term homoeoprophylaxis study in children in North America. Part Two: Safety of HP, review of immunological responses, and effects on general health outcomes.

Free and Healthy Children International HP Research Study-2009-2018.

Keywords: Adverse Events, Children's Health, Developing Immune Systems, Healthy Immunological Response, Immunity, Homoeoprophylaxis (HP), Infectious Disease, Nosodes, Public Health Program, Unvaccinated, Vaccines, Vaccination.

By Kate Birch, RSHom (NA), CCH, Su Sandon, RPh, RSHom (NA), CCH, HMC, Sarah Damlo C. Hom, and Kim Lane, MD.

Abstract

Introduction: The immunological response stimulated by infectious disease develops immunity. Childhood infectious diseases, when naturally contracted, gradually activate and mature immune systems. Both vaccination and the use of nosodes* for homoeoprophylaxis (HP)** aim to introduce infectious agents to activate disease-specific immunological responses and avoid possible risks of natural disease.[lxxi,lxxii,lxxiii] Both methodologies attenuate (weaken) the viral or bacterial agents to minimise the potential risk of too strong an immune system response.[lxxiv] While vaccination comes with attended risks that sometimes are more violent than the actual disease,[lxxv] HP offers a low-risk immunisation method as demonstrated by the production of mild, short-lived immunological responses as the desired response, and improved general health outcomes.

Method: Both unvaccinated and previously vaccinated children registered in a 44-month program to determine the disease specific immunological effects of HP and general health outcomes. Individual responses to the respective nosodes/remedies were documented. Initial and follow-up health profiles tracked ongoing and final health status.

Results: Of the 682 registered children, 475 were *Unvaccinated* and 207 were *Previously Vaccinated.* Of the total 339 respondents, 226 were *Unvaccinated* and 113 were *Previously Vaccinated* and had a total of 1,927 previous vaccine-disease doses. A total of 9,333 individual nosodes/remedy doses were given, which elicited 597 immune responses. Common responses included short-lived fevers, coughs, runny noses, restlessness or sleepiness, and perspiration. Zero adverse events*** were reported in both *Unvaccinated* and *Previously Vaccinated* cohorts.

Incidence of general health conditions improved for all who completed the program. *Unvaccinated* and *Previously Vaccinated* children who completed the program within 50-months, when compared to national averages, experienced above average general health and neurological developmental parameters.

Conclusions: Results demonstrate that HP offers both unvaccinated and previously vaccinated children a low risk immunisation method that improves general health outcomes. Improved health outcomes in *Previously Vaccinated* suggests that HP may be of benefit after previous vaccination.

---

* Nosodes are defined by the Food and Drug Administration's (FDA) Homoeopathic Pharmacopoeia of the United States (HPUS) as homoeopathic "attenuations" of pathological organs and/or tissues, causative agents, or disease products from infected individuals, such as discharges, excretions, and secretions.

** HP can be done with either homoeopathic remedies that best correspond to the acute infective symptom presentation such as in the use of Belladonna as the Genus Epidemicus (GE) for scarlet fever, or with the use of nosodes from active disease. This research is using nosodes except for Lathyrus sativus which has historically been used as a GE for polio.[lxxvi]

*** In research of human subjects an adverse event is defined as a death, life-threatening adverse drug or device experience, inpatient hospitalisation or prolongation of existing hospitalisation, a persistent disability/incapacity, or a congenital anomaly/birth defect.[lxxvii]

Introduction

In this homoeoprophylaxis (HP) research we are working to immunise by introducing infectious disease nosodes. We are not studying the Genus Epidemicus model of HP or using HP for specific disease outbreaks. HP is not vaccination nor a substitute for vaccination.

According to infectious disease theory, natural contraction of an infectious agent is by contact with the mucus membranes which in turn activates a beneficial system-wide cell-mediated immunity (T1 response). This immune activity is marked by chill, fever, and discharge which in turn may stimulate the specific antibody responses of humoral immunity (T2 response). Historically there have been documented developmental benefits associated with natural contraction of childhood infectious disease.[lxxviii] Previous research in HP has suggested that HP stimulates a cell-mediated immune response rather than specific immunity.[lxxix]

Homoeopathy is based on the principle of 'like cures like': a pre-existing condition is cured by a medicinal substance that can produce a similar set of symptoms in a healthy person. In order to investigate the symptom presentation of any substance in a proving we must observe the symptoms that manifest after ingestion of that substance. Homoeopathic Materia Medica volumes list toxicological and proving effects of natural substances.

Furthermore, depending on the child and previous susceptibilities, the kind of response generated can either be a similar response, as in a curative response ('Like Cures Like' for an existing susceptibility), or a dissimilar response that will pass once it has acted out leaving the original susceptibility unchanged.[lxxx] In the case of similar responses, as acute diseases are understood to be a vent for chronic disease,[lxxxi] this mild immunological expression can be seen as an acute disease vent. Improved general health outcomes would indicate that the use of nosodes in this way would prevent the development of chronic disease.

The homoeopathic nosodes used in this HP Program include those made from whooping cough, mumps, measles, pneumonia, meningococcal disease, tetanus, and Haemophilus influenzae type B. Lathyrus sativus, a plant remedy with historical success in the prevention and treatment of polio was used for polio.[lxxxii][lxxxiii] To a greater or lesser extent, fever, perspiration, development of mucus discharge, eruption, or diarrhea may be elicited by one or more of these nosodes mimicking the normal elimination pathway for that disease. In the case of disease specific immunological responses, later exposure to disease will re-activate that immunological memory.[lxxxiv] As crude and potentized infectious agents emit the same frequency it is possible that HP will generate the same immunity that natural exposure would.[lxxxv] The key to the successful development of immunity is in determining what is the sufficient exposure dose of infectious agents. With the appropriate dose, the aim is to stimulate immunity without risk and improve positive general health outcomes.

Research Questions

1. Does HP activate immunological responses and do these responses differ in *Unvaccinated* and *Previously Vaccinated* children?
2. Are these responses proving (dissimilar) responses or healing responses?
3. Does long-term HP improve general health outcomes?
4. How do general health outcomes after HP compare to National rates?
5. What specific HP activated responses are generated?

Method

All children were registered under the supervision of a homoeopathic practitioner trained in HP (HP Supervisor) between April 1, 2009 to December 31, 2014. Once enrolled, they were to undertake a 44-month self-administered HP program, preferably within 50 months, according to a previously set schedule for eight different diseases (see Prophylaxis Record following). At registration an Initial Health Profile and indication of the number of vaccines previously given, if any, outlined the initial health of the child. Study design was based in part on the research by Dr. Isaac Golden.[lxxxvi]

Each child was equipped with:

1. An HP Program Booklet which included the Prophylaxis Record and HP Supervisor contact information.
2. A written comprehensive overview of the program.
3. Written instructions on how to complete the program.
4. A remedy dose/response journal.
5. Three questionnaires to be submitted at three different stages of the program.
6. An HP remedy kit. All nosodes/remedies in the kit were procured from the same registered homoeopathic pharmacy. Sources of nosodes were serologically verified; all nosodes used were procured from active diseases in children collected between 2008 -2011 by San Diego Pathologists.[lxxxvii]

Parameters of Research

For complete parameters of research and informed consent process see Long-term homoeoprophylaxis study in children, Part One: Contributing factors to the successful completion of sequential dosing of disease nosodes.[lxxxviii]

1. **Recruitment**: Passive registration through word of mouth, website searches,[lxxxix] and public lectures.
2. **Data protection**: Publication of the data removes all personal identification of subjects except for the following:
    1. Age.
    2. Geographical subdivisions such as state, province, or country.
    3. General health outcomes and nosode/remedy responses.
3. **Control and Ethical Considerations**: In the study of infectious disease it is unethical to deliberately expose study participants to infectious agents. Therefore, the control group used is infectious disease incidence in vaccinated and unvaccinated populations in the general public.
4. **Blinding**: There was no blinding method built into the study. All participants received the actual nosodes (or in the case of polio, Lathyrus sativus).
5. **Standardisation of Treatment**: All subjects adhered to the HP program as delineated in Chart A. Prophylaxis Record, with dosing dates, was designated for the first Sunday of each month. Adjustment of the program was possible if other needs of the child arose, such as, but not limited to, the following:
    1. If there was an outbreak of a disease covered later in the program, that nosode/remedy could be administered earlier in the program.

2. Supplemental nosodes could be added to the program in case of travel or disease outbreak. Responses to these remedies were not included in this data.

3. If the child was sick at the time when a dose was to be taken, the dosing was postponed until one week after the sickness resolved. The following dose was to be given on time. If the parent forgot to give a dose, they were to give it as soon as they remembered and then continue with the program as scheduled on the first Sunday of the month. They were to wait at least two weeks from the last HP dose before the next disease was introduced.

4. If the parent gave one or two doses of the triple dose and forgot to give the second or third dose, they were instructed to give the entire triple doses series as soon as they remembered.

6. **Data collection**: All data generated was procured directly from the parents via passive submission of follow-up questionnaires. Call for submissions was announced through newsletters, email correspondence, and telephone contact.

The questionnaires are as below.

1. **Initial Health Profile** parameters include:
   1. Gender and age of child at registration
   2. Previous vaccination
   3. Previous infectious disease exposure and acquisition
   4. Initial and ongoing health profiles
   5. General health
      a) Ear infections
      b) Colds/sore throats/coughs
      c) Seasonal allergies
      d) Food allergies
      e) Asthma
      f) Eczema
   6. Behavioral conditions
      g) Violence
      h) Mood swings
      i) Fears
   7. Learning disorders
      j) Speech delay
      k) Disturbance in cognitive function
      l) Disturbance in social function
      m) Neurological conditions

2. **Nosode/Remedy Dosing and Documentation**: All nosode/remedy responses to be logged in the Remedy Journal provided.

7. **Cohorts identified in the following tables**: (numbers and definitions) (200C and 10M denote homoeopathic potency). Potencies selected were based on Isaac Golden's Long-term Homoeoprophylaxis Study:[xc]

1. **Total registered**: Registered with an HP Supervisor by submitting informed consent form, initial health profile, and socio-economic data.

2. *No contact*: No follow-up paperwork was received, or the paperwork was sent and lost in the mail.

3. *Withdrew*: Submission of written notice of withdrawal from the program. Some may have given 1-3 doses before withdrawing.

4. *Started and Stopped*: A few doses in the first series were given and for a variety of reasons they stopped. They did not formally withdraw from the program but provided verbal or written notice of cessation of the program.

5. *200C Series*: Completion of the first 16 months of the program as documented by submission of the first questionnaire and/or Prophylaxis Record.

6. ***200C and first 10M series:*** Completion of the first 16 months and second 8 months of the program as documented by submission of the first and second questionnaires and/or Prophylaxis Record.
7. ***Completed:*** Completion of all stages of the program as documented by submission of the first, second, and third questionnaires and/or Prophylaxis Record.
8. ***Completed in 50 months:*** Completion of the 44-month program within 50 months by comparison of start dates and completion dates documented on questionnaires and/or Prophylaxis Record.
9. ***Unvaccinated:*** Children who had no prior vaccines to registration and remained unvaccinated.
10. ***Previously Vaccinated:*** Children who had received some or all recommended vaccines prior to registration.

8. **Adverse Events:** An Adverse Event reporting procedure was developed to track any life-threatening or permanently disabling events.[xci] Remedy responses that mimic the normal symptoms of the disease are not considered adverse events but rather a proving-like immunological response. Responses that lasted more than 12-24 hours were reviewed and supported with additional dosing or if needed treated homoeopathically based on symptom presentation.

Monthly Doses	Remedy	Potency	Label	Date	Initials	Check for response
1 month	Pertussin	200C	A1			
2 months	Pertussin	200C, 200C, 200C	A1			
3 months	Pneumococcinum	200C	B1			
4 months	Pneumococcinum	200C, 200C, 200C	B1			
5 months	Lathyrus sativus	200C	C1			
6 months	Lathyrus sativus	200C, 200C, 200C	C1			
7 months	Haemophilus (Hib)	200C	D1			
8 months	Haemophilus (Hib)	200C, 200C, 200C	D1			
9 months	Meningococcinum	200C	E1			
10 months	Meningococcinum	200C, 200C, 200C	E1			
11months	Tetanus Toxin	200C	F1			
12 months	Tetanus Toxin	200C, 200C, 200C	F1			
13 months	Parotidinum	200C	H1			
14 months	Parotidinum	200C, 200C, 200C	H1			
15 months	Morbillinum	200C	I1			
16 months	Morbillinum	200C, 200C, 200C	I1			
17 months	Rest or Supplemental Program					
Submit first questionnaire						

Monthly	Remedy	Potency	Label	Date	Initials	Response
18 months	Pertussin	10M, 10M, 10M	A3			
19 months	Pneumococcinum	10M, 10M, 10M	B3			
20 months	Lathyrus sativus	10M, 10M, 10M	C3			
21 months	Haemophilus (Hib)	10M, 10M, 10M	D3			
22 months	Meningococcinum	10M, 10M, 10M	E3			
23 months	Tetanus Toxin	10M, 10M, 10M	F3			
24 months	Parotidinum	10M, 10M, 10M	H3			
25 months	Morbillinum	10M, 10M, 10M	I3			
26 months	Rest or Supplemental Program					
Submit second questionnaire						

Monthly	Remedy	Potency	Label	Date	Initials	Response
28 months	Pertussin	10M, 10M, 10M	A3			
30 months	Pneumococcinum	10M, 10M, 10M	B3			
32 months	Lathyrus sativus	10M, 10M, 10M	C3			
34 months	Haemophilus (Hib)	10M, 10M, 10M	D3			
36 months	Meningococcinum	10M, 10M, 10M	E3			
38 months	Tetanus Toxin	10M, 10M, 10M	F3			
40 months	Parotidinum	10M, 10M, 10M	H3			
42 months	Morbillinum	10M, 10M, 10M	I3			
44 months	Rest or Supplemental Program					
Submit third and final questionnaire						

Chart A. Homoeoprophylaxis program (Prophylaxis Record)

Date of administration to be noted for each dose and check marks for responses which were to be noted in separate journal pages. "One (1) month" is either the age of the child at onset of the program or the first month of doses given.

Remedy relationships: *Pertussin* – Whooping Cough; ***Pneumococcinum*** – Pneumococcus; ***Lathyrus sativus*** – Polio; ***Haemophilus*** – Haemophilus influenzae Type B/Hib; ***Meningococcinum*** – Meningococcus; ***Tetanus toxin*** – Tetanus; ***Parotidinum*** – Mumps; ***Morbillinum*** – Measles

Results

There are four main areas of study summarised in the following tables:

1. Number of *Unvaccinated* and *Previously Vaccinated* registrants, total registrants, and levels of completion in the HP program.
2. Number of doses administered, responses recorded, and adverse events reported in *Unvaccinated* and *Previously Vaccinated* cohorts.
3. General health outcomes of *Completed Unvaccinated* and *Previously Vaccinated* respondents compared to National rates of similar parameters.
4. Common and unique symptoms recorded for each nosode/remedy dosed.

Table 1.1.c. gives numbers and percentages of *Unvaccinated* and *Previously Vaccinated* cohorts at levels of completion in the program; 66.7% of respondents were *Unvaccinated*; 72.2 % of those that completed and 75.8% of those *Completed in 50 months* were unvaccinated.

	Unvaccinated	Previoulsly vaccinated	Totals
1. Total registered	475	207	682
Percentage of total	69.6	30.4	100.0
2. No contact	243	100	343
Percentage of total	70.8	29.2	100.0
Total respondants	226	113	339
Percentage of total repondents	66.7	33.3	100.0
3. Withdrew	21	13	34
Percentage of repondents	61.8	38.2	100.0
4. Started and Stopped	49	22	71
Percentage of repondents	69.0	31.0	100.0
5. 200C series	42	27	69
Percentage of repondents	60.9	39.1	100.0
6. 200C and 10M	23	16	39
Percentage of repondents	59.0	41.0	100.0
7. Completed	91	35	126
Percentage of repondents	72.2	27.8	100.0
8. Completed in 50 months	47	15	62
Percentage of completed	75.8	24.2	100.0

Table 1.1.c. Totals of *Unvaccinated* and *Previously Vaccinated* at all levels of completion

The data for Tables 2.1.a. through to 2.1.f. comes from Prophylaxis Records submitted from 170 out of 339 total respondents. There were 234 respondents who completed some level of the program (cohorts 5, 6, and 7). Not all respondents submitted their Prophylaxis Record, not all dosing series of each nosode/remedy were administered, and not all responses were described. All responses were tallied, regardless of level of completion, if they had check-marked a response.

For each nosode/remedy there are four possible dosing series: 200C single dose, 200C triple dose, and two series of the 10M triple dose. One child may experience several symptoms per dosing series. One dose is 1-3 pellets. There are a total of 10 possible individual doses. Three doses given in twenty-four hours activates one possible immune response. Whether they had one or ten symptoms this is marked as one child with one response.

Table 2.1.a shows the total number of dosing series and actual doses administered compared to the number of responses per each dosing series given. 3,971 total dosing series and 9,333 actual doses were administered. 15.03% of all dosing series produced a response. 35 of the 126 who responded as *Completed* did not provide a Prophylaxis Record, so their number of doses and responses are not included in these tallies. Accordingly, 140 dosing series and 350 individual doses, are not included in these figures as that data was not verified.

	# of dosing series recorded	# of individual doses	# of responses recorded	% of responses for all series
Totals	3971	9333	597	15.03

Table 2.1.a. Total number of nosode/remedy responses as compared to dosing series recorded

Table 2.1.b. reviews reported adverse events compared to the total number of HP dosing series per individual nosode/remedy. As per table 2.1.a., in a total of 9,333 individual doses given, there were no adverse events reported, as defined by the National Institute of Health guidelines for research on human subjects.[xcii]

	# of dosing series given	# of individual of doses	Adverse events reponrted
Pertussin	529	1255	0
Pneumococcinum	510	1204	0
Lathyrus sativus	497	1173	0
Haemophilus (Hib)	487	1145	0
Meningococcinum	490	1146	0
Tetanus Toxin	484	1130	0
Parotidinum	486	1140	0
Morbillinum	488	1140	0

Table 2.1.b. Adverse events reported

Table 2.1.c. shows the total number of *Unvaccinated* and *Previously Vaccinated* children with descriptive symptoms per nosodes/remedy given. This table does not show which vaccines the *Previously vaccinated* had. There were 57 *Unvaccinated* and 22 *Previously Vaccinated* with recorded symptoms. Together these children produced 44.4 % of the total number (#) of check marked responses (265/597). 38 *Unvaccinated* produced symptoms to **Haemophilus** while only 7 *Previously vaccinated* produced symptoms. Of all nosodes **Haemophilus** produced the most responses in *Unvaccinated* (34%) while **Pertussin** produced the most in *Previously Vaccinated*

	Unvaccinated	Previoulsy Vaccinated	Totals
Total respondents	57	22	79
percentage	72.2	27.8	100.0
Total descriptive responses	195	70	265
percentage	73.6	26.4	100.0
1. Pertussin	34	18	52
percentage	65.4	34.6	100.0
2. Pneumociccnum	33	13	46
percentage	71.7	28.3	100.0
3. Lahtyrus	18	9	27
percentage	66.7	33.3	100.0
4. Haemophilus	38	7	45
percentage	84.4	15.6	100.0
5. Meningiococcinum	20	8	28
percentage	71.4	28.6	100.0
6. Tetanus toxin	16	5	21
percentage	76.2	23.8	100.0
7. Parotidinum	18	3	21
percentage	85.7	14.3	100.0
8. Morbillinum	18	7	25
percentage	72.0	28.0	100.0

Table 2.1.c. Total number of *Unvaccinated* and *Previously Vaccinated* respondents with documented symptoms per nosode/remedy

Table 2.1.d. identifies the total number of children experiencing a specific number of nosode/remedy responses based on submitted Prophylaxis Records. 170 records were submitted. Not all doses of all remedies for records submitted were given. There are four dosing sequences of eight diseases. Three doses given in one day activates one possible immune response. The total number of responses any child could possibly have is 4 x 8 = 32. For example, nine children had three total responses from all dosing series. 17.1% of the children only had one response for the entire program. 20 children had two responses which represents 6.7% of the total responses. 14 children produced six total responses representing 14.1% of the total responses. In the 3,971 dosing series recorded, from the 170 Prophylaxis records submitted (from table 2.1.a), a total of 45 children (26.5%) did not have any responses.

# of recorded responses for entire program	0	1	2	3	4	5	6	7	8	9	10	11	12	13	14	15	22	Totals
# of children per # of response	45	29	20	10	15	4	14	6	8	3	6	3	2	2	1	0	2	170
Percentage	26.4	17.0	11.8	5.9	8.8	2.4	8.2	3.5	4.7	1.8	3.5	1.8	1.2	1.2	0.6	0.0	1.2	100.0
Total responses	0	29	40	30	60	20	84	42	64	27	60	33	24	26	14	0	44	597
Percentage	0.0	4.9	6.7	5.0	10.1	3.4	14.0	7.0	10.7	4.5	10.1	5.5	4.0	4.4	2.3	0.0	7.4	100

Table 2.1.d. Total number of responses to nosodes/remedies for the entire program

Table 2.1.e. shows how many responses there were for each dosing series without identifying the nosode/remedy. This table reflects which dosing series stimulated immunological responses more often. For example, 38.4% of the total responses reported occurred during the triple dose of 200C.

	200C	200C x 3	10M x 3	10M x 3	Total responses
Total # of responses per series	197	229	105	66	597
Percentage of total responses	33.0	38.3	17.6	11.1	100.0

Table 2.1.e. Total number of responses per dosing series

Table 2.1.f. identifies the number of dosing series given, individual doses, and the number of responses per dosing series for each nosode/remedy given for all cohorts. Diseases are listed in the order outlined in the program. As there were 69 respondents who only completed the 200C Series more doses of 200C and the triple 200C were recorded for all remedies. The percentage of responses to doses administered should remain constant regardless of sample size. Most children followed the recommended schedule of remedies (Chart A). Not all remedies were given in the order outlined. In cases of possible disease exposure or lifestyle choices the order of remedies may have changed. For example, children going to horse riding camp over summer holidays were recommended to take *Tetanus toxin* out of order; during the measles outbreak in 2014, *Morbillinum* was recommended. There was a total of 529 dosing series (1255 individual doses) of *Pertussin* recorded. 26.09% of the dosing series of *Pertussin* given stimulated a response. This nosode produced the highest percentage of responses of all nosodes. 31.93% were stimulated by the first 200C dose, while 30.49% were stimulated by the triple 200C.

	# of dosing series given	# of individual doses	# of responses recorded	% of responses per series
Pertussin	529	1255	138	26.09%
200C	166	166	53	31.93
200C, 200C, 200C	164	492	50	30.49
10M, 10M, 10M	120	360	23	19.17
10M, 10M, 10M	79	237	12	15.19
Pneumococcinum	510	1204	97	19.02%
200C	163	163	38	23.31
200C, 200C, 200C	164	492	39	23.78
10M, 10M, 10M	111	333	11	9.91
10M, 10M, 10M	72	216	9	12.50
Lathyrus	497	1173	69	13.88%
200C	159	159	19	11.95
200C, 200C, 200C	158	474	30	18.99
10M, 10M, 10M	108	324	10	9.26
10M, 10M, 10M	72	216	10	13.89
Haemophilus (Hib)	487	1145	75	15.40%
200C	158	158	21	13.29
200C, 200C, 200C	156	468	29	18.59
10M, 10M, 10M	105	315	13	12.38
10M, 10M, 10M	68	204	12	17.65

	# of dosing series given	# of individual doses	# of responses recorded	% of responses per series
Meningococcinum	490	1146	60	12.24%
200C	162	162	19	11.73
200C, 200C, 200C	158	474	23	14.56
10M, 10M, 10M	104	312	10	9.62
10M, 10M, 10M	66	198	8	12.12
Tetanus Toxin	484	1130	49	10.12%
200C	161	161	16	9.94
200C, 200C, 200C	157	471	16	10.19
10M, 10M, 10M	104	312	11	10.58
10M, 10M, 10M	62	186	6	9.68
Parotidinum	486	1140	49	10.08%
200C	159	159	14	8.81
200C, 200C, 200C	159	477	19	11.95
10M, 10M, 10M	102	306	11	10.78
10M, 10M, 10M	66	198	5	7.58
Morbillinum	488	1140	60	12.30%
200C	162	162	19	11.73
200C, 200C, 200C	157	471	20	12.74
10M, 10M, 10M	105	315	16	15.24
10M, 10M, 10M	64	192	5	7.81

Table 2.1.f. Total # of responses recorded and # individual doses as compared to # of dosing series given

Table 2.2.a (facing page) pulls data from Table 2.2.b and compares frequency of conditions of those who *Completed in 50 Months* in *Unvaccinated* and *Previously Vaccinated* cohorts, to national incidence data of each condition studied. The national data is collected from studies that took place approximately halfway through the time frame of the research 2009-2018 (half of the registrants entered the program in 2014; entrance closed December 31, 2014). National incidence data for violence, fears, and mood swings is not referenced. 33.30% *Previously Vaccinated* had ear infections upon registration. Incidence dropped to 13.30% by the completion of the program whereas National incidence was 57.8% or between 30%-80%. Incidence of eczema was higher in registrants than national incidence. In *Unvaccinated* incidence rose from 17.0%-19.1% while in *Previously Vaccinated* it dropped from 33.3% to 26.7%. Disturbance in social function in *Previously Vaccinated* rose from 13.3% to 13.6% but remained less than the 20% national rate reported in 2006.

Summary of table 2.2.a: Learning disorders in *Completed in 50 Months*.

3.a. Speech delay: 40% national, 6.4% *Unvaccinated*, and 0% in *Previously Vaccinated*.

3.b. Cognitive dysfunction: 15.4% national, 8.5% *Unvaccinated* and 6.7% *Previously Vaccinated*.

3.c. Social dysfunction: 20% national, 10.6% *Unvaccinated*, and 13.6% *Previously Vaccinated*.

3.d. Neurological conditions: 10.7% national, 4.3% *Unvaccinated*, and 4.5% *Previously Vaccinated*.

	Unvaccinated registrants prior to HP	Unvaccinated HP recipents *Completed* in 50 months	*Previously Vaccinated* registrants prior to HP	Previously Vaccinated HP recipents *Completed* in 50 months	National incidence	Date	Title	Web link
1. General health								
a) Ear infections	10.60%	19.10%	33.30%	13.30%	57.8% 30%-80%	2016 2017	1. Ear Infection and Its Associated Risk Factors in First Nations and Rural School-Aged Canadian Children. 2. Otitis Media in Fully Vaccinated Preschool Children in the Pneumococcal Conjugate Vaccine Era.	https://www.ncbi.nlm.nih.gov/pmc/articles/PMC4764758/ https://www.ncbi.nlm.nih.gov/pmc/articles/PMC5751904/
b) Colds/sore throats/coughs	1 per year 40.4% 2 per year 21.3%	1 per year 12.8% 2 per year 48.9%	1 per year 26.7% 2 per year 26.7% 3 per year 20.0%	1 per year 27.3% 2 per year 13.3% 3 per year 20.0%	6/year average	2015	Viral aetiology of common colds of outpatient children at primary care level and the use of antibiotics	https://www.ncbi.nlm.nih.gov/pmc/articles/PMC3928210/
c) Seasonal allergies	14.9%	25.5%	26.70%	13.3%	11% 7.6%	2012 2017	1. Allergy: wikipedia 2. Summary Health Statistics: National Health Interview Survey	https://en.wikipedia.org/wiki/Allergy#Epidemiology https://ftp.cdc.gov/pub/Health_Statistics/NCHS/NHIS/SHS/2 017_SHS_Table_C-2.pdf
d) Food allergies: unspecified	23.4%	19.1%	40.0%	33.3%	10%. 6.5%	2014 2017	1. Food Allergy. Epidemiology and Natural History. 2. Summary Health Statistics: National Health Interview Survey	https://www.ncbi.nlm.nih.gov/pmc/articles/PMC4254585/ https://ftp.cdc.gov/pub/Health_Statistics/NCHS/NHIS/SHS/2 017_SHS_Table_C-2.pdf
e) Asthma	2.1%	0.0%	13.3%	13.3%	13% 10.8%	2017 2017	1. Summary Health Statistics: National Health Interview Survey 2. Summary Health Statistics: National Health Interview Survey	https://www.cdc.gov/nchs/fastats/asthma.htm https://ftp.cdc.gov/pub/Health_Statistics/NCHS/NHIS/SHS/2 017_SHS_Table_C-2.pdf
f) Eczema	17.00%	19.10%	33.30%	26.70%	12.97%%	2014	Associations of childhood eczema severity: A US population based study	https://www.ncbi.nlm.nih.gov/pmc/articles/PMC4118692/
2. Behavioral conditions								
a) Violence	12.8%	17%%	20.0%	13.3%			Data not found	
b) Mood swings	29.8%	31.9%	66.7%	40.0%			Data not found	
c) Fears	25.5%	36.2%	53.3%	40.0%			Data not found	
3. Learning disorders								
a) Speech delay	4.30%	6.40%	13.3%	0%	40%	2011	Communication skills in a population of primary school-aged children raised in an area of pronounced social disadvantage	https://onlinelibrary.wiley.com/doi/abs/10.1111/j.1460-6984. 2011.00036.x
b) Disturbance in cognitive function	6.4%	8.5%	13.3%	6.7%	15.04%	2008	Trends in the prevalence of developmental disabilities in US children, 1997-2008.	https://www.ncbi.nlm.nih.gov/pubmed/21606152
c) Disturbance in social function	12.8%	10.6%	13.3%	13.6%	20%	2006	Estimating the Prevalence of Early Childhood Serious Emotional/Behavioral Disorders: Challenges and Recommendations	https://www.ncbi.nlm.nih.gov/pmc/articles/PMC1525276/
d) Neurological conditions	4.30%	4.30%	0.0%	4.5%	10.70%	2013	Hospitalizations of children with neurological disorders in the United States	https://www.ncbi.nlm.nih.gov/pmc/articles/PMC3795828/

Table 2.2.a. General health outcomes of *Unvaccinated* and *Previously Vaccinated* in *Completed in 50 months* compared to National incidence

Tables 2.2.b. - 2.2.d. indicate frequency of each condition from Initial and Final Health Profiles. Frequency is relative to the condition and in relationship to the time frame of the questionnaire. The 200C series takes 16 months to complete, the first 10M series takes eight months, and the final 10M series takes an additional 16 months. Final Health Profiles are submitted at the end of the final 10M series. This table does not tell us the changes in health of one individual child as they move through the program however, it delineates the same children at the beginning and at the end. Total # means number of respondents at each stage of the program and frequency denotes annual incidence of each condition on a scale of 1-5 (no incidences of 5 were documented). As the same parent completed each form, their reference scale remained the same throughout the program. These figures include all age groups of participants.

Table 2.2.b. (facing page) for example, 47 *Unvaccinated* (40.4%) had colds at the frequency of 1 upon registration. Whereas the frequency of 1 dropped to 12.8% upon completion but frequency of 2 increased to 48.9%. In the *Previously Vaccinated* frequency of colds at 1 remained the same from the Initial Health Profile to Final Health Profile (26.7%).

Table 2.2.c. (following page) compares Initial and Final Health Profiles outcomes of all *Unvaccinated* and *Previously Vaccinated* registrants who *Completed*. 126 participants completed the program. *50 of them Completed in 50 Months* (see table 2.2.a above). 82 of the 126 who completed submitted the final health questionnaires. Overall, as per the totals or frequency (1-4 frequency) in *Completed* incidence decreased in all conditions except mood swings, fears, and neurological conditions (all three of the neurological conditions we identified as not related to the HP program).

Numbers of children and frequency of said condition.	Initial Health Profile for *Unvaccinated* who completed in 50 months					Total with	Total #	Final Health Profile for *Unvaccinated* who completed program in 50 months					Total with	Total #	Initial Health Profile for *Previously Vaccinated* who completed in 50 months					Total with	Total #	Final Health Profile for *Previously Vaccinated* who completed program in 50 months					Total with	Total #
1. General health	**0**	**1**	**2**	**3**	**4**	**1-4**	**All**	**0**	**1**	**2**	**3**	**4**	**1-4**	**All**	**0**	**1**	**2**	**3**	**4**	**1-4**	**All**	**0**	**1**	**2**	**3**	**4**	**1-4**	**All**
a) Ear infections	42	4	0	1	0	5	47	38	7	1	1	0	9	47	10	5	0	0	0	5	15	13	1	1	0	0	2	15
Percentage	89.36	8.51	0.00	2.13	0.00	10.64	100.00	80.85	14.89	2.13	2.13	0.00	19.15	100.00	66.67	33.33	0.00	0.00	0.00	33.33	100.00	86.67	6.67	6.67	0.00	0.00	13.33	100.00
b) Colds/sore throats/coughs	12	19	10	5	1	35	47	14	6	23	3	1	33	47	2	4	4	3	2	13	15	6	4	2	3	0	9	15
Percentage	25.53	40.43	21.28	10.64	2.13	74.47	100.00	29.79	12.77	48.94	6.38	2.13	70.21	100.00	13.33	26.67	26.67	20.00	13.33	86.67	100.00	40.00	26.67	13.33	20.00	0.00	60.00	100.00
c) Seasonal allergies	40	6	1	0	0	7	47	35	5	6	1	0	12	47	11	2	1	0	1	4	15	13	0	2	0	0	2	15
Percentage	85.11	12.77	2.13	0.00	0.00	14.89	100.00	74.47	10.64	12.77	2.13	0.00	4.30	100.00	73.33	13.33	6.67	0.00	6.67	26.67	100.00	86.67	0.00	13.33	0.00	0.00	13.33	100.00
d) Food allergies	36	2	3	1	5	11	47	38	3	0	0	6	9	47	9	0	4	0	2	6	15	10	1	3	0	1	5	15
Percentage	76.60	4.26	6.38	2.13	10.64	23.40	100.00	80.85	6.38	0.00	0.00	12.77	19.15	100.00	60.00	0.00	26.67	0.00	13.33	40.00	100.00	66.67	6.67	20.00	0.00	6.67	33.33	100.00
e) Asthma	46	0	1	0	0	1	47	47	0	0	0	0	0	47	13	1	1	0	0	2	15	13	1	1	0	0	2	15
Percentage	97.87	0.00	2.13	0.00	0.00	2.13	100.00	100.00	0.00	0.00	0.00	0.00	0.00	100.00	86.67	6.67	6.67	0.00	0.00	13.33	100.00	86.67	6.67	6.67	0.00	0.00	13.33	100.00
f) Eczema	39	4	2	1	1	8	47	38	6	2	0	1	9	47	10	4	0	1	0	5	15	11	3	1	0	0	4	15
Percentage	82.98	8.51	4.26	2.13	2.13	17.02	100.00	80.85	12.77	4.26	0.00	2.13	19.15	100.00	66.67	26.67	0.00	6.67	0.00	33.33	100.00	73.33	20.00	6.67	0.00	0.00	26.67	100.00
2. Behavioral conditions	**0**	**1**	**2**	**3**	**4**	**1-4**	**All**	**0**	**1**	**2**	**3**	**4**	**1-4**	**All**	**0**	**1**	**2**	**3**	**4**	**1-4**	**All**	**0**	**1**	**2**	**3**	**4**	**1-4**	**All**
a) Violence	41	5	1	0	0	6	47	39	6	1	1	0	8	47	12	1	0	0	2	3	15	13	2	0	0	0	2	15
Percentage	87.23	10.64	2.13	0.00	0.00	12.77	100.00	82.98	12.77	2.13	2.13	0.00	17.02	100.00	80.00	6.67	0.00	0.00	13.33	20.00	100.00	86.67	13.33	0.00	0.00	0.00	13.33	100.00
b) Mood swings	33	4	6	2	2	14	47	32	4	7	2	2	15	47	5	3	1	4	2	10	15	9	3	1	2	0	6	15
Percentage	70.21	8.51	12.77	4.26	4.26	29.79	100.00	68.09	8.51	14.89	4.26	4.26	31.91	100.00	33.33	20.00	6.67	26.67	13.33	66.67	100.00	60.00	20.00	6.67	13.33	0.00	40.00	100.00
c) Fears	35	8	0	2	2	12	47	30	6	4	4	3	17	47	7	3	1	2	2	8	15	9	3	3	0	0	6	15
Percentage	74.47	17.02	0.00	4.26	4.26	26.63	100.00	63.83	12.77	8.51	8.51	6.38	36.17	100.00	46.67	20.00	6.67	13.33	13.33	53.33	100.00	60.00	20.00	20.00	0.00	0.00	40.00	100.00
3. Learning disorders	**0**	**1**	**2**	**3**	**4**	**1-4**	**All**	**0**	**1**	**2**	**3**	**4**	**1-4**	**All**	**0**	**1**	**2**	**3**	**4**	**1-4**	**All**	**0**	**1**	**2**	**3**	**4**	**1-4**	**All**
a) Speech delay	45	1	1	0	0	2	47	44	1	1	0	1	3	47	13	2	0	0	0	2	15	15	0	0	0	0	0	15
Percentage	95.74	2.13	2.13	0.00	0.00	4.26	100.00	93.62	2.13	2.13	0.00	2.13	6.38	100.00	86.67	13.33	0.00	0.00	0.00	13.33	100.00	100.00	0.00	0.00	0.00	0.00	0.00	100.00
b) Disturbance in cognitive	44	1	0	2	0	3	47	43	2	0	2	0	4	47	13	1	1	0	0	2	15	14	1	0	0	0	1	15
Percentage	93.62	2.13	0.00	4.26	0.00	6.38	100.00	91.49	4.26	0.00	4.26	0.00	8.51	100.00	86.67	6.67	6.67	0.00	0.00	13.33	100.00	93.33	6.67	0.00	0.00	0.00	6.67	100.00
c) Disturbance in social function	41	2	3	1	0	6	47	42	2	1	1	1	5	47	13	1	1	0	0	2	15	13	1	1	0	0	2	15
Percentage	87.23	4.26	6.38	2.13	0.00	12.77	100.00	89.36	4.26	2.13	2.13	2.13	10.64	100.00	86.67	6.67	6.67	0.00	0.00	13.33	100.00	86.67	6.67	6.67	0.00	0.00	13.33	100.00
d) Neurological conditions	45	0	0	1	1	2	47	45	0	0	0	2	2	47	15	0	0	0	0	0	15	14	1	0	0	0	1	15
Percentage	95.74	0.00	0.00	2.13	2.13	4.26	100.00	95.74	0.00	0.00	0.00	4.26	4.26	100.00	100.00	0.00	0.00	0.00	0.00	0.00	100.00	93.33	6.67	0.00	0.00	0.00	6.67	100.00

Table 2.2.b. Comparison of Initial and Final Health Profiles of *Unvaccinated* and *Previously Vaccinated* who *Completed in 50 months*.

Number of both Unvaccinated and Previoulsy Vaccinated that *Completed* and frequency of said condition.	Frequency upon registration: Initial health profile.					Total 1-4	Total #	Frequency upon complete program: Third and final questionarre.					Total 1-4	Total #
1. General health	0	1	2	3	4	1-4		0	1	2	3	4	1-4	All
a) Ear infections	101	22	2	1	0	25	126	69	10	1	1	1	13	82
Percentage	80.16	17.46	1.59	0.79	0.00	100.00	100.00	84.15	12.20	1.22	1.22	1.22	100.00	100.00
b) Colds/sore throats/coughs	41	44	36	5	0	85	126	10	18	40	12	2	72	82
Percentage	32.54	34.92	28.57	3.97	0.00	100.00	100.00	12.20	21.95	48.78	14.63	2.44	100.00	100.00
c) Seasonal allergies	103	16	4	0	3	23	126	63	6	10	2	1	19	82
Percentage	81.75	12.70	3.17	0.00	2.38	100.00	100.00	76.83	7.32	12.20	2.44	1.22	100.00	100.00
d) Food allergies	99	4	10	3	10	27	126	63	7	4	0	8	19	82
Percentage	78.57	3.17	7.94	2.38	7.94	100.00	100.00	76.83	8.54	4.88	0.00	9.76	100.00	100.00
e) Asthma	122	2	2	0	0	4	126	79	1	1	0	1	3	82
Percentage	96.83	1.59	1.59	0.00	0.00	100.00	100.00	96.34	1.22	1.22	0.00	1.22	100.00	100.00
f) Eczema	106	10	4	2	4	20	126	69	8	3	0	2	13	82
Percentage	84.13	7.94	3.17	1.59	3.17	100.00	100.00	84.15	9.76	3.66	0.00	2.44	100.00	100.00
2. Behavioral conditions	0	1	2	3	4	1-4		0	1	2	3	4	1-4	
a) Violence	108	9	4	2	3	18	126	67	11	2	2	0	15	82
Percentage	85.71	7.14	3.17	1.59	2.38	100.00	100.00	81.71	13.41	2.44	2.44	0.00	100.00	100.00
b) Mood swings	92	11	12	6	5	34	126	45	12	13	10	2	37	82
Percentage	73.02	8.73	9.52	4.76	3.97	100.00	100.00	54.88	14.63	15.85	12.20	2.44	100.00	100.00
c) Fears	93	19	3	6	5	33	126	44	18	9	7	4	38	82
Percentage	73.81	15.08	2.38	4.76	3.97	100.00	100.00	53.66	21.95	10.98	8.54	4.88	100.00	100.00
3. Learning disorders	0	1	2	3	4	1-4		0	1	2	3	4	1-4	
a) Speech delay	118	4	2	2	0	8	126	79	1	1	0	1	3	82
Percentage	93.65	3.17	1.59	1.59	0.00	100.00	100.00	96.34	1.22	1.22	0.00	1.22	100.00	100.00
b) Disturbance in cognitive function	120	3	1	2	0	6	126	76	3	1	2	0	6	82
Percentage	95.24	2.38	0.79	1.59	0.00	100.00	100.00	92.68	3.66	1.22	2.44	0.00	100.00	100.00
c) Disturbance in social function	114	5	5	2	0	12	126	77	0	3	1	1	5	82
Percentage	90.48	3.97	3.97	1.59	0.00	100.00	100.00	93.90	0.00	3.66	1.22	1.22	100.00	100.00
d) Neurological conditions	125	0	1	0	0	1	126	79	0	0	0	3	3	82
Percentage	99.21	0.00	0.79	0.00	0.00	100.00	100.00	96.34	0.00	0.00	0.00	3.66	100.00	100.00

Table 2.2.c. Comparison of Initial and Final Health Profiles of *Unvaccinated* and *Previously Vaccinated* who *Completed*.

Table 2.3. summarises the documented "common symptoms" to all nosode/remedy responses. These responses can be considered proving responses; they lasted for 12-48 hours in most cases. As the substances given (except for Lathyrus) are made from infectious agents most of the proving symptoms are considered "common symptoms" as opposed to "strange, rare, and peculiar (SRP)" symptoms of the immune system expression. The common symptoms of acute disease processes are sleepiness, fever, discharge, and perspiration, etc. There are no modalities, intensity, or frequency noted. (Note these symptoms are not adverse events but the desired mild, short-lived, immune responses that demonstrate immune system engagement with the dosing series.)

Symptoms	
Generals	Cold-like symptoms. Body aches. Restless. Flu-like Symptoms. Exhaustion.
Mind	Irritable. Clingy, cranky, fussy. Oversensitive. Emotional outbursts
Nose	Runny nasal discharge. Nasal congestion. Sneezing.
Throat	Sore throat.
Stomach	Loss of appetite.
Respiratory	Coughing.
Sleep	Tired. Need for sleep. Increase in sleep. Increased sleepiness. Restless during sleep.
Temperature	Fever. High fever. Slight fever. Low-grade fever.

Table 2.3. "Common symptom" nosode/remedy responses

Tables 2.3.1. – 2.3.8. list the unique symptoms (SRP) and some modalities to each nosode/remedy. When combined with the common symptoms above, we can identify the pace, character, and intensity of the normal immunological process of each disease/nosode for clinical indications on homoeopathic practice.

1. Unique Pertussin proving symptoms	
Generals	Uncomfortable. Sanguine. Drained feeling.
Mind	Crabby. Tearful. Fussiness.
Head	Headache.
Face	Flushed cheeks. Dark under eyes.
Eye	Sore eyes.
Nose	Excessive sneezing. Yellow mucous.
Mouth	Increased saliva.
Throat	Scratchy throat. Throat pain when coughing.
Stomach	Spitting up.
Rectum	Runny stools.
Respiratory	Mild coughing. Dry cough. Coughing before bed. Waking at 3 am with coughing. Raspy breathing. Bilateral lung congestion. Chest tightness.
Sleep	Disturbed sleep. Refusal to nap. Crying on waking. Crying on waking.
Temperature	Hot to the touch.
Persiration	Excessive sweating during night.
Skiin	Redness. General mild rash. Red rash on trunk of body and head spreading to arms.

Table 2.3.1. Unique symptoms elicited from Pertussin

2. Unique Pneumococcinum proving symptoms	
Mind	Agitated. Fussiness. Changeable mood. Crying during sleep.
Head	Headache.
Face	Flushed cheeks.
Throat	Scratchy throat.
Nose	Green nasal discharge. Sneezing. Epistaxis.
Mouth	Sore on uppper lip.
Throat	Sore throat. Hoarseness in voice.
Sleep	Fighting sleep.
Skin	Rash.
Respiratory	Mucous producing cough.

Table 2.3.2. Unique symptoms elicited from Pneumococcinum

3. Unique Lathyrus proving symptoms	
Generals	Agitated. Restlessness at night. Disorientation. Signs of discomfort.
Mind	Clingy. Irritable. Lack of focus. Crying during sleep. Sensitive to reprimand.
Nose	Nasal discharge profuse, thick, stringy, clear in color. Epistaxis.
Ear	Ear pain.
Face	Cheeks bright red. Flushed cheeks. Facial blemishes.
Rectum	Runny stool.
Respiratory	Sticky phlegm.
Extremities	Leg pain.
Sleep	Excessive sleeping. Increased sleepiness. Restless during sleep. Frequent waking during sleep.
Temperature	Cold to touch.
Perspiration	Sweaty during sleep.
Skin	Rash on buttocks.

Table 2.3.3. Unique symptoms elicited from Lathyrus sativus

4. Unique Haemophilus proving symptoms	
Generals	Exhaustion, lethargy, fatigue.
Mind	More snuggly. Fussiness. Changeable mood. Whiny, crabby, cranky, weepy. Crying. Very agitated. Night terrors. Doesn't want to follow rules or listen.
Face	Flushing and red patches on face.
Eyes	Green lacrimation from eyes.
Ear	Ear pain.
Nose	Green nasal discharge.
Throat	Neck pain.
Respiratory	Whooping cough-like sypmtoms.
Temperature	Warm trunk.
Skin	Rash, rash on neck, diaper rash. Hives on arms, legs, and face.

Table 2.3.4. Unique symptoms elicited from Haemophilus

Long-term homeoprophylaxis study in children in North America: Part two

5. Unique Meningococcinum proving symptoms	
Generals	Restlessness. Difficulty nursing in children. Teething. Exhaustion. Feeling of being drained.
Face	Facial blemishes.
Stool	Diarrhea.
Sleep	Red spots on belly, arms, and legs.

Table 2.3.5. Unique symptoms elicited from Meningococcinum

6. Unique Tetanus toxin proving symtoms	
Generals	Difficulty nursing in children. Teething. Fidgety behavior. Moving head and eyes around.
Mind	Behavioral changes.
Sleep	Excessive sleeping. Restless in sleep.
Temperature	High fever. Flushed skin with fever.
Skin	General rash on torso and back.

Table 2.3.6. Unique symptoms elicited from Tetanus toxin

7. Unique Parotidinum proving symptoms	
Mind	Irritable. Whiny. Defiant.
Throat	Foul-smelling breath.
Nose	Epistaxis.
Stomach	Decreased appetite. Nausea.
Skin	Rash with small red bumps on upper chest, left side.

Table 2.3.7. Unique symptoms elicited from Parotidinum

8. Unique Morbillinum proving symptoms	
Mind	Irritable. Clingy, cranky. Emotional outbursts. Oversensitive. Hyperactivity.
Throat	White spots on throat.
Stomach	Loss of appetite. Vomiting. Stomach cramps. Stomach ache in morning. Nausea. Vomiting. Better from vomiting.
Rectum	Increase in stool. Loose stool. Diarrhea.

Table 2.3.8. Unique symptoms elicited from Morbillinum

Discussion

1. Number of Unvaccinated and Previously vaccinated and levels of completion. Table 1.1.c:

Ratios between both groups fluctuate with levels of completion. There is an increased percentage of *Unvaccinated* in those *Completed* and *Completed in 50 months*. Whereas the ratio of *Previously Vaccinated* respondents increased in those who stopped at the *200C series* and *200C and 10M series*. These results suggest parents of *Unvaccinated* are more likely to complete a program of HP. From Part One 34% of respondents were under 12 months of age and 66.7% of respondents were *Unvaccinated*.[xciii]

2. Number of doses administered, and responses noted in *Unvaccinated* and *Previously Vaccinated* cohorts compared to adverse events reported. Tables 2.1.a through 2.1.f.

Pertussin produced the highest percentage of responses, 26.09% of all doses and 31.93% of the first dose of 200C. ***Pneumococcinum*** was second in number of responses induced. In all series, except ***Pertussin***, the triple dose of 200C incurred a higher percentage of responses than the single 200C. In all nosodes/remedy responses the first 10M series produced less of a response than the 200Cs, with the final 10M series inducing the least. By the end of the program nosode/remedy responses averaged to between 10-12%. The trend of all dosing series (table 2.1.e.) indicates that as the child moves through the program, as the potency increases, and as the child matures, immune system responses decrease suggesting a reduce in susceptibility to all nosodes/remedies with more doses given.

The only discrepancy to this trend was a "measles outbreak" originating in Los Angeles in 2014, which prompted many to initiate the ***Morbillinum*** series out of order. In this case, the role of age of child and position in the dosing sequence does not correlate. As this program recommends the listed nosode/remedy order we are not able to determine if we would get the same decline in response rate after the first doses when given in a different order: i.e. are the increased responses to ***Pertussin*** and ***Pneumococcinum*** because of the nature of these disease in infants and young children or because they are the first ones given, or both.

3. General health outcomes of *Completed Unvaccinated* and *Previously Vaccinated* respondents compared to national rates of similar parameters. Tables 2.2.a. – 2.2.c.

Incidences of three health categories were recorded in the Initial and Final Health Profiles of *Unvaccinated* and *Previously Vaccinated* cohorts.

1) Physical immune health: acute infective processes of ear infections and colds vs. chronic immune conditions such as seasonal and food allergies, asthma, and eczema.
2) Emotional and behavioral health: violence, mood swings, and fears: reviewing trends in normal behavioral development.
3) Social, cognitive, and neurological function: studying trends in neurological development.

Before and after completion of HP incidences of ear infections and colds in both *Unvaccinated* and *Previously Vaccinated* cohorts were considerably below national incidences. Increases in incidence of both conditions in *Unvaccinated* can be explained by the aging trend of *Unvaccinated* from infants to toddlers. Infants, under one year of age, have fewer ear infections and colds than toddlers.[xciv] In *Previously Vaccinated* ear infection incidence dropped through the HP program as these children grew out of ear infection age (2-5). Seasonal allergies follow this same course confirming that allergies are uncommon in infants but more common as children age. However, the incidence drops in *Previously Vaccinated*, suggesting that HP might lower susceptibility to seasonal allergies.

Asthma and eczema are normally rare or non-existent in infants for the first 6 months of life. Of the older children, who had either, incidence stayed the same or went down as the program progressed. At registration incidence of these were higher than national incidence signifying a discrepancy between actual incidence in our cohort and national reported incidence. A five-year follow-up is needed to determine if long-term health outcomes continued in this trajectory.

Before and after HP frequency of violence, mood swings, and fears increased in *Unvaccinated* where these same conditions decreased in *Previously Vaccinated*. One explanation for this could be that most of the unvaccinated were infants at the beginning of the program where incidence of these conditions was low to non-existent and children grew into these conditions. *Previously Vaccinated* included older children who, as they proceeded through the program, grew out of these conditions. In both cohorts these changes most likely had nothing to do with HP.

While mood swings, fears, and sometimes violence may be normal as children grow and develop their personalities the same cannot be said for speech delay, cognitive and social dysfunction, or neurological conditions, as per the following comparisons for both cohorts *Completed* with national rates. Results also show on all levels *Unvaccinated* had less incidence than *Previously Vaccinated* and all children who participated in HP had less incidence than national rates. Rates of each condition are slightly higher in those *Completed in 50 months*. Due to a small sample size, explanations for this cannot be drawn.

Of the three children who developed neurological conditions categorised at the frequency of 4 in *Unvaccinated* two were over 10 years old upon registration, one had Down Syndrome and the other was previously diagnosed with Asperger's and OCD by the age of seven. The third was also over 10 years old and developed migraines. In these cases, the process of HP had little to do with their development or mitigation of neurological conditions.

4.   **Common and unique symptoms recorded for each nosode/remedy dosed.**

Tables 2.3.1-2.3.8 list the Materia Medica of seven nosodes and Lathyrus sativus. Table 2.3.1. records common symptoms and does not list descriptive symptomatology or modalities. The common symptoms reported are typical of cell-mediated immune response. Unique symptoms can be used to differentiate the homoeopathic indications of these nosodes/remedies and normal immune responses from HP. Out of 261 children who indicated responses, 175 developed only 1-2 responses during the entire program but nearly all children showed improvement in general health outcomes indicating that there can be improved health outcomes even if immunological responses are not generated, suggesting that HP nosodes can act curatively to previous susceptibilities. Furthermore, responses of *Unvaccinated Previously Vaccinated* were similar, demonstrating that some previous vaccines did not detrimentally affect the kind of responses generated.

None of the responses induced posed risk or detrimental long-term health consequences to the participants.

Conclusions

Long-term homoeoprophylaxis is a low risk method of immunisation alternative which activates mild, short-lived immune system responses which improves general health outcomes for both *Unvaccinated* and *Previously Vaccinated* children. Repeated dosing produces fewer responses demonstrating a reduced susceptibility of the recipient to subsequent dosing.

When compared to national averages, children who utilise HP are less likely to develop chronic health conditions. These results suggest HP induced immune responses may help to reduce incidence of chronic health conditions. The most significant outcome is that learning disorders and neurological issues do not develop and remain next to nil throughout the entire HP program. This, when compared to national averages of the general population, clearly establishes that HP recipients experienced improved general health outcomes that exceed current national averages.

Economic disclosure

Sponsored by Free and Healthy Children International (FHCi). 612-338-1668 FHCint@gmail.com https://freeandhealthychildren.org/

1. Principle Investigator: Kate Birch, RSHom, CCH, 612-701-0629, katebhom@hotmail.com
2. Document Collection Person: Su Sandon, RPh, RSHom (NA), CCH, HMC, 612-889-2683 suhomeopathy@earthlink.net
3. Medical Advisor: Kim Lane, MD, 651-347-1952 wellnesslane@comcast.net

Data Entry:

4. Sarah Damlo, 952-212-3372, FHCigrants@gmail.com
5. Tana Harahan, 651-272-0932, FHCint@gmail.com
6. Katie Bromme, 612-327-3855, FHCiresearch@gmail.com
7. Max Sagert, 651-587-4047, FHCiresearch@gmail.com

Who	Total paid from 2009-2019 (USD)
Kate Birch	$4,815.00
Su Sandon	$6,865.77
Sarah Damlo	$3,885.00
Katie Bromme	$1,466.25
Max Sagert	$1,011.50
Tana Harahan	$670.00
Kim Lane	N/A
Total paid	$18,713.52

Free and Healthy Children International (FHCi) is a 501(c)3 non-profit membership organisation dedicated to research, education, and access to homoeoprophylaxis. It is registered for business in the state of MN, USA. From April 2009-December 2014, 682 children were registered in this research. From January 2015 to July 16, 2019 we did not have a tracking system in place. Since July 17, 2017, to September 2019 an additional 1,044 children registered with FHCi.

We are independently funded by individual contributions and membership dues. All fees paid for organising and tabulating the research were dispersed on either a quarterly stipend or hourly basis. There are no personal direct economic benefits derived from the results of this study. FHCi is not economically associated with any pharmacy that would benefit from the sale of the homoeopathic remedies utilised in this research. All research staff are homoeopaths and live in the state of MN. We did this research because we are invested in the health of children. Thank you to everyone who helped this research come to fruition. Homoeoprophylaxis is for free and healthy children!

References*

*Reference numeration continues from previous section.

l.   Birch, K (2014). Vaccines and homoeoprophylaxis share the same history. https://freeandhealthychildren.org/2014/03/16/vaccines-and-homeoprophylaxis-history/ (Last viewed 4 October 2019).

li.   Hahnemann, S. "The Cure and Prevention of Scarlet Fever." Lessor Writings. B Jain Publishers, New Delhi.

lii.   Castro, D., Nogueira, G (1968). "Use of the nosode Meningococcinum as a preventative against meningitis." Journal of the American Institute of Homeopathy. 4 (Dec.): 211-219.

liii.   Plitnick, L (2013). Global regulatory guidelines for vaccines. Nonclinical development of novel biologics, biosimilars, vaccines and specialty biologics. https://www.sciencedirect.com/topics/neuroscience/attenuated-vaccine (Last viewed 4 October 2019)

liv.   Pertussis (whooping cough) disease and vaccine quick facts. National Vaccine Information Center. https://www.nvic.org/vaccines-and-diseases/whooping-cough/quick-facts.aspx (Last viewed 4 October 2019)

lv.   Sheffield, F (2014). Homeoprophylaxis: Human Records, Studies and Trials. https://www.homeopathycenter.org/news/homeoprophylaxis-human-records-studies-and-trials

lvi.   (1999). Guidance on reporting adverse events to institutional review boards for NIH-supported multicenter clinical trials. National Institute of Health. US. https://grants.nih.gov/grants/guide/notice-files/not99-107.html (Last viewed 4 October 2019)

lvii.   Adams, D (2018). Rudolf Steiner on Traditional Childhood Illnesses and Vaccines. https://paam.wildapricot.org/resources/Pictures/07%20RS-Traditional%20Childhood%20Illnesses%20and%20Vaccines.pdf (Last viewed 4 October 2019)

lviii.   Bracho, G (2013). "Homeoprophylaxis: Evidences from Basic Research and Practical Applications." Homeopathy Research Institute, Barcelona.

lix.   Hahnemann, S (1997). The Organon of Medicine. 5th Edition translated by Dudgeon. 6th Edition translated by Boericke. Paragraphs 34-40. http://www.homeopathyhome.com/reference/organon/organon.html (Last viewed 4 October 2019)

lx.   Hahnemann, S (1991). The Chronic Diseases. New Delhi: B. Jain Publishers.

lxxxii.   Sheffield, F (2014). Homeoprophylaxis: Human Records, Studies and Trials. https://www.homeopathycenter.org/news/homeoprophylaxis-human-records-studies-and-trials) (Last Viewed 4 October 2019).

lxi.   Janeway, C., Travers, P., Walport, M., Shlomchik, M (2001). Immunological memory. Garland Science. New York. https://www.ncbi.nlm.nih.gov/books/NBK27158/ (Last viewed 4 October 2019).

lxii.   Montagnier, L (2009). Electromagnetic Signals Are Produced by Aqueous Nanostructures Derived from Bacterial DNA Sequences. Interdiscip Sci Comput Life Sci DOI: 10.1007/s12539-009-0036-7. http://sphq.org/wp-content/uploads/2016/03/etudes_Montagnier_Electro-signals-produced-by-aqueous-DNA.pdf (Last viewed 4 October 2019)

lxiii.   Golden, I (2004). The Potential Value of Homeoprophylaxis in the Long-Term Prevention of Infectious Diseases, and the Maintenance of General Health in Recipients. Graduate School of Integrative Medicine Swinburne University of Technology. https://immunizationalternatives.com/wp-content/uploads/2015/04/HP_Isaac_Golden_thesis_homeoprophylaxis1.pdf (Last viewed 4 October 2019)

lxiv.   San Diego Pathologists. Certificate of Analysis. https://freeandhealthychildren.org/certification-in-homeoprophylaxis/hpdocuments/remedy-sources/ (Last viewed 4 October 2019).

lxv.   Birch, K, Sandon, S, Damlo, S, Lane, K (2019). Long-term homeoprophylaxis study in children, part one: Contributing factors to the successful completion of sequential dosing of disease nosodes. Similia; Journal for the Australian Society of Homeopaths. Australia.

lxvi.   Free and Healthy Children International (FHCi). 612-338-1668 FHCint@gmail.com

lxvii.   Golden, I (2004). Potential Value of Homoeoprophylaxis in the Long-Term Prevention of Infectious Diseases, and the Maintenance of General Health in Recipients. Graduate School of Integrative Medicine Swinburne University of Technology. https://immunizationalternatives.com/wp-content/uploads/2015/04/HP_Isaac_Golden_thesis_homeoprophylaxis1.pdf (Last viewed 4 October 2019).

lxviii.   (1999). Guidance on reporting adverse events to institutional review boards for NIH-supported multicenter clinical trials. National Institute of Health. US. https://grants.nih.gov/grants/guide/notice-files/not99-107.html (Last viewed 4 October 2019)

lxix.   Ibid.

lxx.   Birch, K, Sandon, S, Damlo, S, Lane, K (2019). Long-term homeoprophylaxis study in children in North America, part one: Contributing factors to the successful completion of sequential dosing of disease nosodes. Similia; Journal for the Australian Society of Homeopaths. Australia.

lxxi.   Saurabh, M, Neha, G, Swathi, S, Shefali, K, Yekaternia, S (2017). Otitis Media in Fully Vaccinated Preschool Children in the Pneumococcal Conjugate Vaccine Era. Glob Pediatr Health. 2017; 4: 2333794X17749668 https://www.ncbi.nlm.nih.gov/pmc/articles/PMC5751904/. (Last viewed 4 October 2019).

4. Appendix

The following are additional tables not included in the published Part Two. Coding of numbers are as follows. The tables in Part Two are registered with 2.1, 2.2, 2.3. etc. based on the topic they are summarizing. Within each grouping there may be sub-tables such as 2.2.a., 2.2 b. etc. The tables listed below, as in, 3.2.2. f. etc. are appendix tables in continuation of the respective series in Part Two.

These tables all summarize relevant data for our research, but for conciseness in the published papers, were not included in the official results.

Table 3.2.1.a.i. (following page) reflects the number of children who had documented 1-2, 3-4, 5-6, or 7-8 out of 8 possible responses per dosing series. There were a total of 8 possible doses per series (each triple dose series is called one dose) and a total of 32 possible doses and responses for each child if they completed the entire program and responded to every dose in all dosing series. If there was a response during the 0-48 hours after dosing either the single or the triple dosing series, or if there were multiple symptoms expressed, one response was tallied. In some instances, children took more doses than required if they had gotten sick with a random disease at the time of initial dosing whereby the nosode was repeated, if there was a prolonged response to the dose to mitigate that response, or if there was a possible exposure to the disease. We only tallied the doses and responses during completion of the recommended schedule.

Each child submits one prophylaxis record. In that record, if they indicated a response to each dose given in a particular dosing series there would be a value placed in the 7-8 responses row. For example, 2 children had 7-8 responses to the single 200C dosing series. 1 had 7-8 out of 8 possible responses to the triple 200C series and one had 7-8 responses to the triple 200C, and another child had 7-8 responses to the first 10M series. For the single 200C series recorded, 60 children had 1-2 responses out of 8 possible responses while 62 children had 1-2 responses to the triple 200C.

This table does not indicate if the same children who had 1-2 responses to the first 200C had 1-2 responses to the triple 200C. Nor, if the child who had 7-8 responses to the 200C triple dose or was one of the two children who had 7-8 responses to the single 200C dose.

There was a total of 261 recorded responses to all doses regardless of nosode/remedy given. 1-2 responses were recorded 85 times from the single 200C dose, 98 times for the triple 200C, 48 times for the first 10M series, and 30 times for the second 10M. As this table does not specify the children who responded it does not indicate the maximum number of responses a specific child may have had for the duration of the program. Table 2.1.d. (Part Two) indicates the how many children had how many responses. The top number of recorded responses for one child was 22 and there were two children who had 22 responses. See Table 2.1.f (Part Two) for the nosode/remedy specific number of responses to doses recorded.

Not all children who submitted questionnaires for all of levels of completion submitted prophylaxis records. All prophylaxis records were sourced for number of responses regardless of level of completion of program.

	200C	200C x 3	10M x 3	10M x 3	Total recorded responses
Total recorded repsonses of each series	85	98	48	30	261
1 - 2 responses	60	62	33	20	175
Percentage of total 1 - 2 responses	34.3	35.4	18.9	11.4	100.0
3 - 4 responses	15	28	12	4	59
Percentage of total 3 - 4 responses	25.4	47.5	20.3	6.8	100.0
5 - 6 responses	8	7	2	6	23
Percentage of total 5 - 6 responses	34.8	30.4	10.6	52.5	128.3
7 - 8 responses	2	1	1	0	4
Percentage of total 7 - 8 responses	50.0	25.0	4.9	0.0	79.9

Table 3.2.1.a.i. Number of children with recorded number of responses from each dosing series

Table 3.2.2.d. (facing page) compares the health profiles of the same *Unvaccinated* children upon registration and completion. 81.8% of children had no ear infections upon completion while 90.2% did upon registration. All incidence of colds, seasonal allergies, increased through the course of the program while food allergies, asthma and eczema dropped by 1-2 children during the program. It is normal for children to have some incidence of seasonal colds in childhood. It is common for seasonal allergies to develop after 2-3 years of life. As many of the *Unvaccinated* were infants upon registration, this increase can be attributed to the aging of the children. The same is true for violence, mood swings, and fears to normally appear from age 2-3 on.

Asthma and eczema are not normally occurring in unvaccinated children in the general population. These numbers reflect this trend. This in comparison to same *Previously Vaccinated* children who completed (see Table 3.2.2.g. below) is an example of how, in general, unvaccinated children are healthier in these parameters than vaccinated children.

In all learning disorder categories, there was a 1-5% decrease in incidence in the *Unvaccinated* who *Completed*. Specifics on these conditions in these children was not captured.

Insidence of said condition in the Unvaccinated Registrants who Completed	Frequency upon registration: Initial health profile.						Total #	Frequency upon complete program: Third and final questionarre.						Total #
1. General health	0	1	2	3	4	1-4		0	1	2	3	4	1-4	
a) Ear infections	74	7	1	0	0	82	82	68	12	1	1	0	14	82
Percentage	90.2	8.5	1.2	0.0	0.0	9.8	100.0	82.9	14.6	1.2	1.2	0.0	17.1	100.0
b) Colds/sore throats/coughs	40	21	15	5	1	42	82	25	15	37	4	1	57	82
Percentage	48.8	25.6	18.3	6.1	1.2	51.2	100.0	30.5	18.3	45.1	4.9	1.2	69.5	100.0
c) Seasonal allergies	74	7	1	0	0	8	82	65	7	8	1	1	17	82
Percentage	90.2	8.5	1.2	0.0	0.0	9.8	100.0	79.3	8.5	9.8	1.2	1.2	20.7	100.0
d) Food allergies	70	2	4	2	4	12	82	71	3	1	0	7	11	82
Percentage	85.4	2.4	4.9	2.4	4.9	14.6	100.0	86.3	3.7	1.2	0.0	8.5	13.4	100.0
e) Asthma	81	0	1	0	0	1	82	81	0	0	0	1	1	82
Percentage	98.8	0.0	1.2	0.0	0.0	1.2	100.0	98.3	0.0	0.0	0.0	1.2	1.2	100.0
f) Eczema	70	5	2	1	4	12	82	72	6	2	0	2	10	82
Percentage	85.4	6.1	2.4	1.2	4.9	14.6	100.0	87.8	7.3	2.4	0.0	2.4	12.2	100.0
2. Behavioral conditions	0	1	2	3	4	1-4		0	1	2	3	4	1-4	
a) Violence	74	5	2	0	1	8	82	69	9	2	2	0	13	82
Percentage	90.2	6.1	2.4	0.0	1.2	9.8	100.0	84.1	11.0	2.4	2.4	0.0	15.9	100.0
b) Mood swings	64	7	7	1	3	18	82	54	9	11	6	2	28	82
Percentage	78.0	8.5	8.5	1.2	3.7	22.0	100.0	65.9	11.0	13.4	7.3	2.4	34.1	100.0
c) Fears	67	12	0	1	2	15	82	50	14	7	6	5	32	82
Percentage	81.7	14.6	0.0	1.2	2.4	18.3	100.0	61.0	17.1	8.5	7.3	6.1	39.0	100.0
3. Learning disorders	0	1	2	3	4	1-4		0	1	2	3	4	1-4	
a) Speech delay	81	0	1	0	0	1	82	79	1	1	0	1	3	82
Percentage	98.8	0.0	1.2	0.0	0.0	1.2	100.0	96.3	1.2	1.2	0.0	1.2	3.7	100.0
b) Disturbance in cognitive function	79	1	0	2	0	3	82	78	2	0	2	0	4	82
Percentage	96.3	1.2	0.0	2.4	0.0	3.7	100.0	95.1	2.4	0.0	2.4	0.0	4.9	100.0
c) Disturbance in social function	75	2	4	1	0	7	82	75	3	2	1	1	7	82
Percentage	91.5	2.4	4.9	1.2	0.0	8.5	100.0	91.5	3.7	2.4	1.2	1.2	8.5	100.0
d) Neurological conditions	77	0	0	1	4	5	82	80	0	0	0	2	2	82
Percentage	93.9	0.0	0.0	1.2	4.9	6.1	100.0	97.6	0.0	0.0	0.0	2.4	2.4	100.0

Table 3.2.2.d. Health Profiles of *Unvaccinated* who *Completed* upon registration and at the end of the program.

Table 3.2.2.e. (facing page) compares frequency of conditions of all *Unvaccinated* at four stages of the program:

1. Registration
2. after completion of the 200C series (First questionnaire)
3. after completion of the 200C triple and first 10M series (Second questionnaire)
4. the Second 10M series (Third and final questionnaire).

Total # refers to the number of children in that stage. For example, 475 *Unvaccinated* registered, 120 submitted the First questionnaire, 87 Submitted the Second, and 82 the Final.

398 of the 475 total registrants (representing 83.8% of the total) *Unvaccinated* had no ear infections upon registration. Of the 82 that completed, 68 (82.9%) had no ear infections. 16.2% of *Unvaccinated* registrants had ear infections to some degree of frequency, while only 17.1% of those that *Completed* had them. While this table shows the total number of children at each stage it does not accurately reflect the change in incidence of the specific children that completed. See Table 3.2.2.d. above.

Appendix

Number of *Unvaccinated* registrants and frequency of said condition.	Frequency upon registration: Initial health profile.						Total #	Frequency after 200C Series: First questionaire.						Total #	Frequency after 200C and first 10M series: Second questionaire.						Total #	Frequency upon complete program: Third and final questionaire.						Total #
1. General health	0	1	2	3	4	1-4		0	1	2	3	4	1-4		0	1	2	3	4	1-4		0	1	2	3	4	1-4	
a) Ear infections	398	67	8	1	1	77	475	97	19	3	0	1	23	120	73	10	3	1	0	14	87	68	12	1	1	0	14	82
Percentage	83.8	14.1	1.7	0.2	0.2	16.2	100.0	80.8	15.8	2.5	0.0	0.8	19.2	100.0	83.9	11.5	3.4	1.1	0.0	16.1	100.0	82.9	14.6	1.2	1.2	0.0	17.1	100.0
b) Colds/sore throats/coughs	181	148	107	33	6	294	475	5	43	62	10	0	115	120	6	38	35	8	0	81	87	25	15	37	4	1	57	82
Percentage	38.1	31.2	22.5	6.9	1.3	61.9	100.0	4.2	35.8	51.7	8.3	0.0	95.8	100.0	6.9	43.7	40.2	9.2	0.0	93.1	100.0	30.5	18.3	45.1	4.9	1.2	69.5	100.0
c) Seasonal allergies	425	36	9	3	2	50	475	100	13	6	1	0	20	120	65	11	10	1	0	22	87	65	7	8	1	1	17	82
Percentage	89.5	7.6	1.9	0.6	0.4	10.5	100.0	83.3	10.8	5.0	0.8	0.0	16.7	100.0	74.7	12.6	11.5	1.1	0.0	25.3	100.0	79.3	8.5	9.8	1.2	1.2	20.7	100.0
d) Food allergies	405	22	19	6	23	70	475	95	8	5	2	10	25	120	73	5	4	2	3	14	87	71	3	1	0	7	11	82
Percentage	85.3	4.6	4.0	1.3	4.8	14.7	100.0	79.2	6.7	4.2	1.7	8.3	20.8	100.0	83.9	5.7	4.6	2.3	3.4	16.1	100.0	86.6	3.7	1.2	0.0	8.5	13.4	100.0
e) Asthma	465	6	3	1	0	10	475	117	1	1	1	0	3	120	86	1	0	0	0	1	87	81	0	0	0	1	1	82
Percentage	97.9	1.3	0.6	0.2	0.0	2.1	100.0	97.5	0.8	0.8	0.8	0.0	2.5	100.0	98.9	1.1	0.0	0.0	0.0	1.1	100.0	98.8	0.0	0.0	0.0	1.2	1.2	100.0
f) Eczema	402	37	13	8	15	73	475	93	15	6	1	5	27	120	71	11	4	0	1	16	87	72	6	2	0	2	10	82
Percentage	84.6	7.8	2.7	1.7	3.2	15.4	100.0	77.5	12.5	5.0	0.8	4.2	22.5	100.0	81.6	12.6	4.6	0.0	1.1	18.4	100.0	87.8	7.3	2.4	0.0	2.4	12.2	100.0
2. Behavioral conditions	0	1	2	3	4	1-4		0	1	2	3	4	1-4		0	1	2	3	4	1-4		0	1	2	3	4	1-4	
a) Violence	435	19	10	6	5	40	475	105	8	5	2	0	15	120	72	8	4	1	2	15	87	69	9	2	2	0	13	82
Percentage	91.6	4.0	2.1	1.3	1.1	8.4	100.0	87.5	6.7	4.2	1.7	0.0	12.5	100.0	82.8	9.2	4.6	1.1	2.3	17.2	100.0	84.1	11.0	2.4	2.4	0.0	15.9	100.0
b) Mood swings	387	32	27	20	9	88	475	71	18	9	14	8	49	120	52	13	8	7	7	35	87	54	9	11	6	2	28	82
Percentage	81.5	6.7	5.7	4.2	1.9	18.5	100.0	59.2	15.0	7.5	11.7	6.7	40.8	100.0	59.8	14.9	9.2	8.0	8.0	40.2	100.0	65.9	11.0	13.4	7.3	2.4	34.1	100.0
c) Fears	373	54	21	19	8	102	475	74	16	11	11	8	46	120	51	13	8	10	5	36	87	50	14	7	6	5	32	82
Percentage	78.5	11.4	4.4	4.0	1.7	21.5	100.0	61.7	13.3	9.2	9.2	6.7	38.3	100.0	58.6	14.9	9.2	11.5	5.7	41.4	100.0	61.0	17.1	8.5	7.3	6.1	39.0	100.0
3. Learning disorders	0	1	2	3	4	1-4		0	1	2	3	4	1-4		0	1	2	3	4	1-4		0	1	2	3	4	1-4	
a) Speech delay	462	4	4	4	1	13	475	113	2	4	1	0	7	120	82	4	0	0	1	6	87	79	1	1	0	1	3	82
Percentage	97.3	0.8	0.8	0.8	0.2	2.7	100.0	94.2	1.7	3.3	0.8	0.0	5.8	100.0	94.3	4.6	0.0	0.0	1.1	5.7	100.0	96.3	1.2	1.2	0.0	1.2	3.7	100.0
b) Disturbance in cognitive function	464	6	2	3	0	11	475	117	1	1	1	0	3	120	82	3	1	0	1	5	87	78	2	0	2	0	4	82
Percentage	97.7	1.3	0.4	0.6	0.0	2.3	100.0	97.5	0.8	0.8	0.8	0.0	2.5	100.0	94.3	3.4	1.1	0.0	1.1	5.7	100.0	95.1	2.4	0.0	2.4	0.0	4.9	100.0
c) Disturbance in social function	453	8	11	3	0	22	475	114	3	0	2	1	6	120	83	1	0	2	1	4	87	76	3	2	1	1	7	82
Percentage	95.4	1.7	2.3	0.6	0.0	4.6	100.0	95.0	2.5	0.0	1.7	0.8	5.0	100.0	95.4	1.1	0.0	2.3	1.1	4.6	100.0	91.5	3.7	2.4	1.2	1.2	8.5	100.0
d) Neurological conditions	463	1	2	3	6	12	475	115	0	0	1	4	5	120	85	0	0	1	1	2	87	80	0	0	0	2	2	82
Percentage	97.5	0.2	0.4	0.6	1.3	2.5	100.0	95.8	0.0	0.0	0.8	3.3	4.2	100.0	97.7	0.0	0.0	1.1	1.1	2.3	100.0	97.6	0.0	0.0	0.0	2.4	2.4	100.0

Table 3.2.2.e. Frequency of Conditions in all *Unvaccinated* at all four stages of the program

Table 3.2.2.f. compares the health profiles of *Previously Vaccinated* upon registration and at the end of the program. In this group you can see 81.8% of children had no ear infections upon completion while 63.6% did upon registration. Colds, seasonal allergies, asthma, increases through the course of the program while violence, mood swings, fears, and speech delay decrease.

The three children that demonstrated an increase in disturbance in cognitive function, disturbance in social function, and neurological conditions had other preexisting conditions specifically, Down's syndrome, autism and migraine headaches, respectively. Otherwise no Learning disorders developed during the program in the *Previously Vaccinated* who *Completed*.

Number of *Previously Vaccinated* children who *Completed* and frequency of said condition.	Frequency upon registration: Initial health profile.						Total #	Frequency upon completion of program: Third and final questionarre.						Total #
1. General health	0	1	2	3	4	1-4		0	1	2	3	4	1-4	
a) Ear infections	14	8	0	0	0	8	22	18	3	0	0	1	4	22
Percentage	63.6	36.4	0.0	0.0	0.0	36.4	100.0	81.8	13.6	0.0	0.0	4.5	18.2	100.0
b) Colds/sore throats/coughs	2	11	5	2	2	20	22	1	6	6	8	1	21	22
Percentage	9.1	50.0	22.7	9.1	9.1	90.9	100.0	4.5	27.3	27.3	36.4	4.5	95.5	100.0
c) Seasonal allergies	18	1	3	0	0	4	22	17	2	2	1	0	5	22
Percentage	81.8	4.5	13.6	0.0	0.0	18.2	100.0	77.3	9.1	9.1	4.5	0.0	22.7	100.0
d) Food allergies	14	1	4	1	2	8	22	14	4	3	0	1	8	22
Percentage	63.6	4.5	18.2	4.5	9.1	36.4	100.0	63.6	18.2	13.6	0.0	4.5	36.4	100.0
e) Asthma	21	1	0	0	0	1	22	20	1	1	0	0	2	22
Percentage	95.5	4.5	0.0	0.0	0.0	4.5	100.0	90.9	4.5	4.5	0.0	0.0	9.1	100.0
f) Eczema	18	4	0	0	0	4	22	18	3	1	0	0	4	22
Percentage	81.8	18.2	0.0	0.0	0.0	18.2	100.0	81.8	13.6	4.5	0.0	0.0	18.2	100.0
2. Behavioral conditions	0	1	2	3	4	1-4		0	1	2	3	4	1-4	
a) Violence	15	3	2	0	2	7	22	19	2	0	1	0	3	22
Percentage	68.2	13.6	9.1	0.0	9.1	31.8	100.0	86.4	9.1	0.0	4.5	0.0	13.6	100.0
b) Mood swings	10	3	3	5	1	12	22	11	5	2	4	0	11	22
Percentage	45.5	13.6	13.6	22.7	4.5	54.5	100.0	50.0	22.7	9.1	18.2	0.0	50.0	100.0
c) Fears	12	5	1	2	2	10	22	13	5	3	1	0	9	22
Percentage	54.5	22.7	4.5	9.1	9.1	45.5	100.0	59.1	22.7	13.6	4.5	0.0	40.9	100.0
3. Learning disorders	0	1	2	3	4	1-4		0	1	2	3	4	1-4	
a) Speech delay	20	2	0	0	0	2	22	21	1	0	0	0	1	22
Percentage	90.9	9.1	0.0	0.0	0.0	9.1	100.0	95.5	4.5	0.0	0.0	0.0	4.5	100.0
b) Disturbance in cognitive function	20	1	1	0	0	2	22	19	1	2	0	0	3	22
Percentage	90.9	4.5	4.5	0.0	0.0	9.1	100.0	86.4	4.5	9.1	0.0	0.0	13.6	100.0
c) Disturbance in social function	20	1	1	0	0	2	22	19	1	2	0	0	3	22
Percentage	90.9	4.5	4.5	0.0	0.0	9.1	100.0	86.4	4.5	9.1	0.0	0.0	13.6	100.0
d) Neurological conditions	22	0	0	0	0	0	22	21	1	0	0	0	1	22
Percentage	100.0	0.0	0.0	0.0	0.0	0.0	100.0	95.5	4.5	0.0	0.0	0.0	4.5	100.0

Table 3.2.2.f. Health Profiles of *Previously Vaccinated* who *Completed* upon registration and at the end of the program.

Table 3.2.2.g. (following page) compares frequency of conditions of all *Previously Vaccinated* at four stages of the program

1. Registration
2. after completion of the 200C series (First questionnaire)
3. after completion of the 200C triple and first 10M series (Second questionnaire)
4. the Second 10M series (Third and final questionnaire).

Total # refers to the number of children in that stage. For example, 207 *Previously Vaccinated* registered, 60 submitted the First questionnaire, 33 Submitted the Second, and 22 the Final.

135 of the 207 total registrants who submitted forms (representing 65.2% of the total) *Previously Vaccinated* had no ear infections upon registration. Of the 22 that completed, 18 (81.8%) had no ear infections. 34.8% of *Previously Vaccinated* registrants had ear infections to some degree of frequency, while only 18% of those that *Completed* had them. While this table shows the total number of children at each stage it does not accurately reflect the change in incidence of the specific children that completed. See Table 3.2.2.f. above.

Number of *Previously Vaccinated* registrants and frequency of said condition	Frequency upon registration: Initial health profile.						Total #	Frequency after 200C Series: First questionairre.						Total #	Frequency after 200C and first 10M series: Second questionaire.						Total #	Frequency upon completion of program: Third and final questionarre.						Total #
1. General health	0	1	2	3	4	1-4		0	1	2	3	4	1-4		0	1	2	3	4	1-4		0	1	2	3	4	1-4	
a) Ear infections	135	57	12	2	1	72	207	46	12	1	1	0	14	60	24	7	2	0	0	9	33	18	3	0	0	1	4	22
Percentage	65.2	27.5	5.8	1.0	0.5	34.8	100.0	76.7	20.0	1.7	1.7	0.0	23.3	100.0	72.7	21.2	6.1	0.0	0.0	27.3	100.0	81.8	13.6	0.0	0.0	4.5	18.2	100.0
b) Colds/sore throats/coughs	26	86	73	20	2	181	207	3	25	25	6	1	57	60	2	14	12	5	0	31	33	1	6	6	8	1	21	22
Percentage	12.6	41.5	35.3	9.7	1.0	87.4	100.0	5.0	41.7	41.7	10.0	1.7	95.0	100.0	6.1	42.4	36.4	15.2	0.0	93.9	100.0	4.5	27.3	27.3	36.4	4.5	95.5	100.0
c) Seasonal allergies	158	30	11	4	4	49	207	47	7	3	1	2	13	60	23	4	4	2	0	10	33	17	2	2	1	0	5	22
Percentage	76.3	14.5	5.3	1.9	1.9	23.7	100.0	78.3	11.7	5.0	1.7	3.3	21.7	100.0	69.7	12.1	12.1	6.1	0.0	30.3	100.0	77.3	9.1	9.1	4.5	0.0	22.7	100.0
d) Food allergies	158	13	8	9	19	49	207	45	3	1	5	6	15	60	21	3	2	1	6	12	33	14	4	3	0	1	8	22
Percentage	76.3	6.3	3.9	4.3	9.2	23.7	100.0	75.0	5.0	1.7	8.3	10.0	25.0	100.0	63.6	9.1	6.1	3.0	18.2	36.4	100.0	63.6	18.2	13.6	0.0	4.5	36.4	100.0
e) Asthma	197	5	4	1	0	10	207	58	0	2	0	0	2	60	32	1	0	0	0	1	33	20	1	1	0	0	2	22
Percentage	95.2	2.4	1.9	0.5	0.0	4.8	100.0	96.7	0.0	3.3	0.0	0.0	3.3	100.0	97.0	3.0	0.0	0.0	0.0	3.0	100.0	90.9	4.5	4.5	0.0	0.0	9.1	100.0
f) Eczema	157	25	10	6	9	50	207	50	6	2	1	1	10	60	27	5	1	0	0	6	33	18	3	1	0	0	4	22
Percentage	75.8	12.1	4.8	2.9	4.3	24.2	100.0	83.3	10.0	3.3	1.7	1.7	16.7	100.0	81.8	15.2	3.0	0.0	0.0	18.2	100.0	81.8	13.6	4.5	0.0	0.0	18.2	100.0
2. Behavioral conditions	0	1	2	3	4	1-4		0	1	2	3	4	1-4		0	1	2	3	4	1-4		0	1	2	3	4	1-4	
a) Violence	166	20	10	8	3	41	207	45	6	5	3	1	15	60	30	3	0	0	0	3	33	19	2	0	1	0	3	22
Percentage	80.2	9.7	4.8	3.9	1.4	19.8	100.0	75.0	10.0	8.3	5.0	1.7	25.0	100.0	90.9	9.1	0.0	0.0	0.0	9.1	100.0	86.4	9.1	0.0	4.5	0.0	13.6	100.0
b) Mood swings	130	24	16	26	11	77	207	28	12	5	9	6	32	60	19	6	3	4	1	14	33	11	5	2	4	0	11	22
Percentage	62.8	11.6	7.7	12.6	5.3	37.2	100.0	46.7	20.0	8.3	15.0	10.0	53.3	100.0	57.6	18.2	9.1	12.1	3.0	42.4	100.0	50.0	22.7	9.1	18.2	0.0	50.0	100.0
c) Fears	128	30	14	27	8	79	207	27	15	4	10	4	33	60	21	7	3	2	0	12	33	13	5	3	1	0	9	22
Percentage	61.8	14.5	6.8	13.0	3.9	38.2	100.0	45.0	25.0	6.7	16.7	6.7	55.0	100.0	63.6	21.2	9.1	6.1	0.0	36.4	100.0	59.1	22.7	13.6	4.5	0.0	40.9	100.0
3. Learning disorders	0	1	2	3	4	1-4		0	1	2	3	4	1-4		0	1	2	3	4	1-4		0	1	2	3	4	1-4	
a) Speech delay	201	3	3	0	0	6	207	55	1	1	0	3	5	60	30	1	0	1	1	3	33	21	1	0	0	0	1	22
Percentage	97.1	1.4	1.4	0.0	0.0	2.9	100.0	91.7	1.7	1.7	0.0	5.0	8.3	100.0	90.9	3.0	0.0	3.0	3.0	9.1	100.0	95.5	4.5	0.0	0.0	0.0	4.5	100.0
b) Disturbance in cognitive function	198	4	2	1	2	9	207	55	2	1	1	1	5	60	32	1	0	0	0	1	33	19	1	2	0	0	3	22
Percentage	95.7	1.9	1.0	0.5	1.0	4.3	100.0	91.7	3.3	1.7	1.7	1.7	8.3	100.0	97.0	3.0	0.0	0.0	0.0	3.0	100.0	86.4	4.5	9.1	0.0	0.0	13.6	100.0
c) Disturbance in social function	189	7	7	3	1	18	207	55	1	2	2	0	5	60	31	1	1	0	0	2	33	19	1	2	0	0	3	22
Percentage	91.3	3.4	3.4	1.4	0.5	8.7	100.0	91.7	1.7	3.3	3.3	0.0	8.3	100.0	93.9	3.0	3.0	0.0	0.0	6.1	100.0	86.4	4.5	9.1	0.0	0.0	13.6	100.0
d) Neurological conditions	202	3	0	0	2	5	207	56	3	0	0	1	4	60	32	1	0	0	0	1	33	21	1	0	0	0	1	22
Percentage	97.6	1.4	0.0	0.0	1.0	2.4	100.0	93.3	5.0	0.0	0.0	1.7	6.7	100.0	97.0	3.0	0.0	0.0	0.0	3.0	100.0	95.5	4.5	0.0	0.0	0.0	4.5	100.0

Table 3.2.2.g. Health profiles of all *Previously Vaccinated* at all four stages of the program.

Tables 3.2.3.1.a. - 3.2.3.8.a. indicate the unique and common symptoms developed in response to each nosode or remedy given in the program. Responses are identified as to which dose, 200C single or triple, or either 10M series, and isolated between *Unvaccinated* and *Previously Vaccinated* cohorts. These symptoms do not identify the subject or if they responded to either or both the 200C and 10M series. We assume not all symptoms were recorded, either due to lack of observational skills on the parent's behalf, or not all details being considered a part of the process. I.e. did the baby wake from a nap in a sweat? Did someone else get the baby and not make note of it? Was that symptom dismissed because it was rationalized for some external reason, etc.?

Many respondents noted there was a response but failed to identify the response. I.e. There were a total of 138 claimed responses to **Pertussin** (Part One, Table 2.1) on the Prophylaxis Records submitted but only 54 total responses were noted. These are listed in the following tables. The number in brackets, e.g., (3), identifies how many times that symptom was noted. I.e., fussiness was noted in response to *Pertussin* from three separate children. These groupings of symptoms represent a Materia Medica of that nosode or remedy and represent a proving of sorts, thus they can be used to register the nosode in the HPUS monograph. These responses are not side-effects but rather immune system responses showing that the immune system is registering the disease and responding in such a way to develop immunity. Also, these symptoms can be used as homeopathic indications for the use of the nosode in practice when a case presents with similar symptoms.

1. Pertussin proving symptoms	200C responses	10M responses
# of unvaccinated respondents	24	12
Generals	Cold-like symptoms. Restless. Fatigue. Uncomfortable.	
Mind	Irritable. Crabby. Tearful. Fussiness (3). Fussiness at night.	Irritable. Emotional (3). Fussy.
Head	Headache.	
Face	Flushed cheeks.	
Eye	Sore eyes.	
Nose	Runny nasal discharge (4). Nasal congestion (2). Sneezing. Excessive sneezing.	Nasal congestion. Runny nasal discharge(3).
Mouth	Increased saliva.	
Throat	Scratchy throat.	
Stomach	Spitting up.	Nausea.
Rectum	Runny stools.	Diarrhea.
Respiratory	Coughing (2). Mild coughing. Dry cough. Coughing before bed. Waking at 3 am with coughing.	Mild cough. Cough (4)
Sleep	Tired (2). Increased sleepiness. Disturbed sleep. Refusal to nap. Restless during sleep. Restlessness at night.	Sleepiness (2). Restless during sleep.
Temperature	Fever (2). Low-grade fever (2). Hot to the touch.	Low-grade fever.
Persiration	Perspiration.	Excessive sweating during night.
Skiin	Redness. General mild rash. Red rash on trunk of body and head spreading to arms.	
# of vaccinated respondents	12	6
Generals	Cold-like symptoms. Restless.Sanguine.	Fatigue. Drained feeling.
Mind	Behavioral changes. Irritable. Fussy.	
Head		Headache.
Face		Dark under eyes.
Nose	Yellow mucous.	Runny nasal discharge. Slight nasal congestion.
Throat	Sore throat. Scratchy throat. Throat pain when coughing.	Sore throat.
Stomach	Decreased appetite.	Stomach upset.
Rectum	Diarrhea.	Loose stool.
Respiratory	Coughing (4). Raspy breathing. Bilateral lung congestion.	Coughing.
Chest	Chest tightness.	
Sleep	Tired. Sleepiness. More sleep than usual. Frequent waking. Crying on waking.	
Temperature		Fever. Low-grade fever.

Table 3.2.3.1.a. Unique and common symptoms in response to Pertussin

2. Pneumococcinum responses	200C responses	10M responses
# of unvaccinated respondents	21	12
Generals	Cold-like symptoms (2). Restless.	Cold-like symptoms (3).
Mind	Irritable (3). Agitated. Fussiness (2). Emotional. Changeable mood. Crying during sleep.	Whiney. Fussiness. Crying
Face	Flushed cheeks.	
Nose	Nasal congestion. Sinus congestion. Runny nasal discharge (6). Green nasal discharge. Sneezing.	Runny nasal discharge (3). Nasal congestion.
Mouth	Sore on uppper lip.	
Throat	Sore throat. Hoarseness in voice (2).	
Stomach		Loss of appetite.
Respiratory	Dry cough.	Cough (2).
Sleep	Tired. Sleepy. Increased sleepiness (2). Fighting sleep.	Sleepiness (2).
Temperature	Fever.	
Skin	Rash.	
# of vaccinated respondents	9	4
Head	Headache.	
Nose	Slight nasal congestion. Epistaxis.	
Throat	Scratchy throat.	
Rectum		Diarrhea. Increase in stool. Runny stool. Loose stool (2).
Respiratory	Coughing. Increase in cough. Mucous producing cough.	
Temperature	Fever.	

Table 3.2.3.2.a. Unique and common symptoms in response to Pneumococcinum

3. Lathyrus responses	200C responses	10M responses
# of unvaccinated respondents	17	6
Generals	Cold-like symptoms. Agitated. Restless. Restlessness at night.	Clingy. Disorientation. Signs of discomfort. Restlessness.
Mind	Irritable (3). Emotional. Lack of focus. Crying during sleep.	Sensitive to reprimand.
Nose	Runny nasal discharge. Nasal congestion. Nasal discharge profuse, thick, stringy, clear in color.	Runny nasal discharge. Nasal congestion.
Ear		Ear pain.
Throat	Soreness in throat.	Cough.
Face	Cheeks bright red (2). Flushed cheeks.	
Stomach	Decrease in appetite.	
Rectum		Runny stool.
Respiratory	Cough (2). Sticky phlegm.	
Sleep	Excessive sleeping. Increased sleepiness (4). Restless during sleep.	Frequent waking during sleep.
Temperature	Low-grade fever. Cold to touch.	Fever.
Skin	Rash on buttocks.	
# of vaccinated respondents	5	4
Face	Facial blemishes.	
Nose	Epistaxis. Stuffy nose.	Nasal congestion.
Rectum		Diarrhea.
Extrmities	Leg pain.	
Sleep		Sleepy.
Temperature	Low-grade fever.	Low-grade fever.
Perspiration	Sweaty during sleep.	

Table 3.2.3.3.a. Unique and common symptoms in response to Lathyrus sativus

4. Haemophilus responses	200C responses	10M responses
# of unvaccinated respondents	25	13
Generals	Restless.	Restless. Flu-like symptoms, achey, exhaustion, lethargy, fatigue.
Mind	More snuggly. Fussiness (2). Changeable mood (2). Whiny (2), crabby, cranky, weepy.	Whiny (2). Crying. Very agitated. Night terrors. Doesn't want to follow rules or listen.
Face	Flushed cheeks.	Flushing and red patches on face.
Eyes	Green lacrimation from eyes.	
Ear	Ear pain.	
Nose	Runny nasal discharge (2). Nasal congestion. Sneezing. Green nasal discharge.	Runny nose (3)
Throat		Sore throat.
Respiratory		Neck pain.
Stomach		Vomiting.
Respiratory	Cough (2), whooping cough-like sypmtoms.	Cough (2).
Sleep	Tired. Sleepy. Excessive sleeping. Increased sleepiness. Restless in sleep.	
Temperature	Fever (3). High fever, low-grade fever (2). Elevated body temperature (2), warm trunk.	Fever (5).
Skin	Rash, rash on neck, diaper rash.	
# of vaccinated respondents	5	2
Mind	Irritable.	
Nose	Runny nasal discharge (3).	
Throat		Sore throat.
Stomach		Stomach ache.
Sleep	Tired. Sleepiness.	
Temperature	Low grade fever.	Fever.
Skin	Hives on arms, legs, and face.	

Table 3.2.3.4.a. Unique and common symptoms in response to Haemophilus influenzae

5. Meningococcinum responses	200C responses	10M responses
# of unvaccinated respondents	15	5
Generals	Restlessness. Difficulty nursing in children. Teething.	Exhaustion.
Mind	Irritable (2). Cranky, fussy.	Whiny. Behavioral changes.
Nose	Runny nose (2).	Runny nasal discharge.
Stomach		Decrease in appetite. Thirsty. Nausea.
Respiratory	Coughing worse at night.	Mild cough.
Sleep	Tired (3). Excessive sleeping. Difficulty sleeping.	Restlessness during sleep. Sleepy (2).
Temperature	High fever.	
Skin	Red spots on belly, arms, and legs.	
# of vaccinated respondents	5	3
Generals	Feeling of being drained.	Feeling of being drained.
Mind	Change in behavior. Slightly fussy. Irritable.	
Nose	Nasal congestion. Runny nasal discharge.	
Face		Facial blemishes.
Rectum		Diarrhea (2).
Temperature	Low-grade fever.	

Table 3.2.3.5.a Unique and common symptoms in response to Meningococcinum

6. Tetanus toxin responses	200C responses	10M responses
# of unvaccinated respondents	8	8
Generals	Restlessness. Difficulty nursing in children. Teething.	Behavioral changes.
Mind	Irritable (2). Cranky, fussy.	Behavioral changes. Whiny.
Nose	Runny nose (2).	Runny nasal discharge.
Respiratory	Coughing worse at night.	Mild cough.
Sleep	Tired (3). Excessive sleeping. Difficulty sleeping.	Sleepy (2). Restlessness during sleep.
Temperature	High fever.	
Skin	General rash on torso and back.	
# of vaccinated respondents	4	1
Generals	Cold-like symptoms. Fidgety behavior. Moving head and eyes around.	Cold-like symptoms.
Mind	Irritable, moody.	Irritable.
Throat	Runny nasal discharge.	Stuffy nose, runny nose (2).
Stomach	Vomiting.	
Respiratory	Coughing (2).	Coughing.
Sleep	Excessive sleeping. Restless in sleep.	
Temperature		Fever (3). Flushed skin with fever. Slight fever. Low-grade fever.
Skin	General rash on torso and back.	

Table 3.2.3.6.a. Unique and common symptoms in response to Tetanus toxin

7. Parotidinum responses	200C responses	10M responses
# of *Unvaccinated* respondents	12	6
Generals	Cold-like symptoms.	
Mind	Irritable (2). Whiny.	
Throat	Sore throat.	Foul-smelling breath.
Nose	Runny nose (2). Sneezing.	Runny nose.
Stomach	Decreased appetite.	Nausea.
Respiratory		Cough.
Sleep	Excessive sleeping. Early waking.	Tired (3).
Temperature	Fever. High fever.	Fever (2). Low-grade fever.
Skin	Rash with small red bumps on upper chest, left side.	
# of vaccinated respondents	2	1
Generals		Fatigue.
Mind	Irritable. Defiant.	
Nose	Epistaxis.	
Sleep	Sleepiness.	
Temperature	Fever.	

Table 3.2.3.7.a. Unique and common symptoms in response to Parotidinum

8. Morbillinum responses	200C responses	10M responses
# of *Unvaccinated* respondents	13	5
Generals	Cold-like symptoms (2).	Cold-like symptoms.
Mind	Irritable. Clingy, cranky.	Oversensitive.
Nose	Runny nose (2). Sneezing.	
Throat	Sore throat. White spots on throat.	
Stomach	Loss of appetite. Vomiting.	Stomach ache in morning. Nausea. Vomiting. Better from vomiting.
Rectum	Increase in stool. Loose stool.	
Respiratory	Coughing (2).	
Sleep	Tired (3). Need for sleep. Increase in sleep. Restless during sleep.	Tired. Sleepy.
Temperature	Slight fever. Low-grade fever. Alternating between hot and cold.	Fever.
# of vaccinated respondents	4	3
Generals	Body aches.	Hyperactivity.
Mind	Emotional outbursts.	
Nose	Runny nose. Congestion in sinus.	
Throat	Sore throat.	Sore throat.
Stomach	Stomach cramps.	Vomiting.
Rectum	Diarrhea.	
Respiratory	Cough (2).	
Sleep	Tired (2). Need for sleep. Restless sleep.	
Temperature	Slight fever.	Fever.

Table 3.2.4. (following page) summarizes the number of children exposed to the specified diseases as compared to contraction rates, degree of suffering in the disease process, how many doses of the nosode or previous vaccines or disease-specific vaccines they had received. Of the 19 children exposed to whooping cough, 7 contracted. Of those who contracted only one had completed all 4 series of the nosode and two had been previously vaccinated with a whooping cough-containing vaccine. The youngest of those who contracted whooping cough was 11 months and severity of symptoms expression was at a level 1. The 5-6 -year-old who had taken all HP doses had level 3 symptom expression. In the cases of children who contracted mumps or measles, did so despite having received both HP for each disease and MMR vaccination. These numbers are insufficient to give any understanding of the efficacy of HP but do warrant further investigation.

This table is not a part of the published papers as the number of children who were exposed versus who contracted were too small to give any significant results. The complexity contraction versus number of doses and previous vaccines warrants further research.

This chart references the scale used for degree of suffering.

	Scale of contracted disease experience
1	Mild: 24 hours or less, Mild or intense symptoms with fast resolution
2	Moderate: symptoms lasting 2-6 days
3	Excessive: symptoms or prolonged lasting 7 or more days
4	Severe: Needed medical intervention

Disease	Number Exposed	Ref. Number	Disease contracted	Degree of suffering (1-4)	Doses of respective nosode completed at time of exposure				Age of Child at time exposure/ contraction	Total # of all vaccine-disease doses	# of doses of disease-specific vaccine-disease previoulsy given
					200C	200C 3X	10M 3X	10M 3X			
Whooping cough	19	1	no		1	1	1	1	unspecified	0	
		2	no		1	1	1	1	unspecified	0	
		3	no		1	1	1	1	2.4 years	0	
		4	no		1	1	1	1	4.1 years	0	
		5	no		1	1			2 years	0	
		6	no		1	1			8.4 years	29	3
		7	no		1	1			6.11 years	31	4
		8	no		1	1			2.10 years	0	
		9	no		1	1			2nd grade	0	
		10	no		1	1			8 months	0	
		11	no		1	1			1.10 years	0	
		12	no		1	1			unspecified	0	
		13	yes	3	1	1	1	1	5.6 years	0	
		14	yes	1	1	1			11 months	0	
		15	yes	2	1	1			4.8 years	13	3
		16	yes	2	1	1			6.10 years	15	4
		17	yes	1	1	1			2.5 years	0	
		18	yes	1	1	1			10 years	0	
		19	yes	1	1	1			1.9 years	0	
Pneumonia	4	1	no		1	1	1	1	3.7 years	0	
		2	no		1	1	1		5.2 years	0	
		3	no		1	1			2.2 years	3	0
		4	yes	4	1	1	1	1	3 years	0	
Polio	0	0							n/a		
Haemophilus (Hib)	0	0							n/a		
Meningitis	0	0							n/a		
Tetanus	0	0							n/a		
Mumps	2	1	no		1	1	1	1	10.1 years	15	2
		2	yes	3	1	1	1	1	7.11 years	13	1
Measles	3	1	no		1	1			8.11 years	29	1
		2	no		1	1			7.6 years	31	1
		3	yes	1	1	1	1	1	3.4 years	0	

Table 3.2.4. Number of children exposed to disease versus contraction rates

 Appendix

Thank you for taking the time to understand HP and the results demonstrated in this study. These numbers are promising and assuring for those looking for options. More research is necessary to expand the access and use of HP.

May all children be free!